Advances in
CATARACT SURGERY

New Orleans Academy of Ophthalmology

Edited by

Glen C. Cangelosi, MD

SLACK Incorporated, 6900 Grove Road, Thorofare, New Jersey 08086

SLACK International Book Distributors

In Canada:
McGraw-Hill Ryerson Limited
330 Progress Avenue
Scarborough, Ontario
Canada MIP 2Z5

In Europe and the United Kingdom:
Simon Kugler Publications bv
P.O. Box 516
1180 Am Amstelveen
The Netherlands

Quest Meridien Ltd.
145a Croydon Road
Beckenham, Kent
England BR3 3RB

In Australia and New Zealand:
MacLennan & Petty Pty Limited
P.O. Box 425
Artarmon, N.S.W. 2064
Australia

In Japan:
Igaku-Shoin Ltd.
Tokyo International
P.O. Box 5063
1-28-36 Hongo, Bunkyo-Ku
Tokyo 113
Japan

In Asia and India:
PG Publishing Pte Limited.
36 West Coast Road, #02-02
Singapore 0512

Foreign Translation Agent

John Scott & Company
International Publishers' Agency
417-A Pickering Road
Phoenixville, PA 19460
Fax: 215-988-0185

Managing Editor: Lynn C. Borders
Production Manager: David Murphy
Publisher: Harry C. Benson

Printed in the United States of America

Library of Congress Catalog Card Number: 89-043616

ISBN 1-55642-164-8

Published by: SLACK Incorporated
              6900 Grove Rd.
              Thorofare, NJ 08086-9447

Last digit is print number: 10 9 8 7 6 5 4 3 2 1

CONTENTS

CONTRIBUTORS

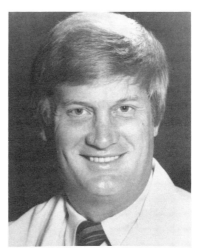

DAVID J. APPLE, MD
Professor and Chairman
Department of Ophthalmology
Medical University of South Carolina
Charleston, South Carolina

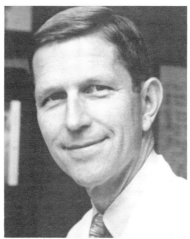

HAL D. BALYEAT, MD
Clinical Professor
Department of Ophthalmology
The University of Oklahoma and
The Dean A. McGee Eye Institute
Oklahoma City, Oklahoma

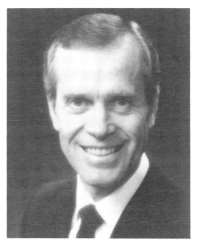

**HOWARD V. GIMBEL, MD,
FRCSC, FAAO**
Clinical Assistant Professor
University of Calgary
Department of Surgery
Calgary, Alberta, Canada

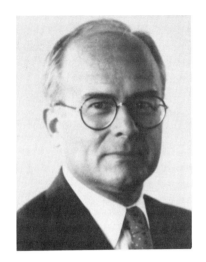

JOHN D. HUNKELER, MD
Clinical Associate Professor
of Ophthalmology
University of Kansas
School of Medicine
Kansas City, Kansas

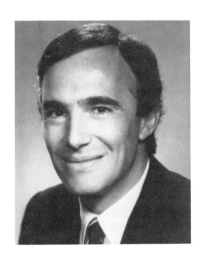

CALVIN W. ROBERTS, MD
Associate Professor of Ophthalmology
Cornell University Medical College
New York, New York

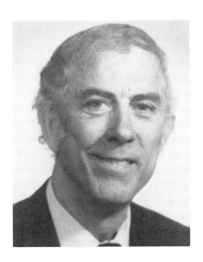

C. WILLIAM SIMCOE, MD
Associate Professor of Ophthalmology
University of Oklahoma
Tulsa Medical College
Tulsa, Oklahoma

PREFACE

Ophthalmology is a fascinating specialty due to its dynamic nature and its quest for perfection. This fact is reflected in the refinement of its surgical techniques and postoperative results. The New Orleans Academy of Ophthalmology has witnessed these changes over the last four decades. For example, in 1978 the NOAO's symposium on cataracts included debates on the differences between intracapsular, extracapsular, and phacoemulsification techniques of cataract extraction. By 1987 the Academy's symposium isolated the debate between extracapsular versus phacoemulsification techniques. The most recently held symposium in 1990 appeared to favor the latest advances in small-incision phacoemulsification and implants. This book represents a compilation of those formal lectures, case presentations, and roundtable discussions presented at the New Orleans Academy of Ophthalmology's 39th Annual Symposium, Advances in Cataract Surgery, held on March 2–4, 1990. Our thanks go to our guest speakers and SLACK, Incorporated for making this book possible.

Glen C. Cangelosi, MD
Editor

Chapter 1

PERIBULBAR ANESTHESIA

Hal D. Balyeat, MD

Retrobulbar anesthesia is a technique which has stood the test of time. Since its initial use by Knapp in 1984,[1] the technique has been used successfully with minor modification. The modern technique was described by Atkinson in 1948.[2] He suggested using procaine hydrochloride (novocaine), 2 percent with epinephrine (1:1,000). Lid akinesia was obtained by the O'Brien method using a 25-gauge needle 2.0 cm. in length. Retrobulbar anesthesia and akinesia was obtained using a rounded point 22-gauge needle, 4.5 cm. in length. A kin wheal was made at the junction of the middle and temporal orbital rim just below the inferior temporal margin of the orbit using a 27-gauge needle injecting a small amount of 2 percent novocaine. The retrobulbar needle was then introduced through the wheal injecting approximately 0.5 cc of anesthetic solution as the needle was introduced into the orbit in an attempt to reduce pain when the orbital septum was pierced. After a short pause the patient was directed to look up and away from the site of the injection as the needle was directed upward and inward, midway between the lateral and inferior rectus muscles. The rationale for this maneuver was to access the muscle cone more easily. It was Atkinson's belief that the fascial sheath of the muscles which close the spaces between the rectus muscles for a little distance back of the globe were moved forward and upward, out of the way, which prevented the needle from striking the fascial extension. After the needle was advanced 2.5 cm to 3.5 cm depending on the size of the orbit, 1 to 1.5 cm. of novocaine was injected slowly, followed by removal of the needle and gentle massage with a rotary motion.

The fact that this technique, with minor variations, is still used by a majority of ophthalmologists 42 years after its description is a tribute to its efficacy and safety.

In 1977, Koornneef demonstrated by orbital dissection and cross-sectional reconstructions of the orbit that the concept of a well-defined muscle cone was inaccurate. He showed that the posterior "intermuscular septum" is poorly defined with only a few connective tissue septa within the muscle cone.[3] In 1981, Unsold et al demonstrated by CT analysis that the traditional upward and inward position of gaze during the administration of retrobulbar anesthesia increased the risk of dural sheath penetration and globe perforation.[4] This is brought about by stretching of the optic nerve with downward and outward displacement. In high myopia, the posterior pole of the eye moves inferiorly which places it in the path of the needle. These two studies, especially the latter, may have sparked renewed interest in anesthesia techniques which have resulted in many of the variations in methods used currently.

Bupivacaine hydrochloride (Marcaine) in ophthalmic surgery was first reported in 1966,[5] and in the American literature in 1974.[6] It was apparent that the increased duration of action was valuable in the reduction of post operative pain. The use of bupivacaine in ophthalmic anesthesia increased dramatically because of this. Coincidentally, an increasing number of complications of retrobulbar anesthesia were reported. Among these were retrobulbar hemorrhage, globe perforation, central retinal artery and vein occlusion.[7-9]

The emergence of ultrasound and CT scanning has helped support the etiologic concepts in many of these cases. More recently, however, respiratory arrest following retrobulbar anesthesia has been reported.[10-13] Smith, in an editorial, implicated bupivacaine as the responsible agent in a number of cases of respiratory arrest which had been reported to him by various surgeons.[14] The exact etiology was unknown, although the possibility of injection into the optic nerve sheath could have occurred. Wittpenn et al prospectively followed 3123 retrobulbar injections given over a one year period by different surgeons at the Wilmer Institute.[13] Approximately two-thirds of the patients received an anesthetic agent consisting of 2% lidocaine and 0.75% bupivacaine (50:50 mixture totalling 10 cc.) while one-third of the patients received a similar agent prepared with 4% lidocaine. Patients receiving 4% lidocaine mixed with bupivacaine had an almost ninefold greater risk of respiratory arrest as compared to the patients receiving 2% lidocaine mixed with bupivacaine (7/888 versus 2/2235).

It was their conclusion that the risk of respiratory arrest following retrobulbar injection was related to the total amount of anesthetic agent placed in the retrobulbar space. According to Grizzard,[15] the most likely cause of respiratory arrest, contralateral amaurosis, and cranial nerve palsies following contralateral injection is intranerve injection of anesthetic with passage of the anesthetic through the subdural space of the nerve into the brainstem. This conclusion is based on studies by Antoszyk and Buckley,[16] Friedbert and Kline,[17] Javitt and coworkers,[18] and Drysdale.[19]

Perhaps as a result of the increasing awareness of complications of retrobulbar anesthesia, renewed interest was demonstrated in anesthesia technique including needle selection and methods of anesthetic administration.

It is a common belief among many ophthalmologists and anesthesiologists that blunt needles are safer than sharp needles. The usual justification for this belief is that it is more difficult to penetrate the globe, optic nerve sheath or blood vessels with a blunt needle. This, unfortunately, is not the case. Grizzard has correctly pointed out that the "increased resistance caused by the blunt needle is not appreciated because of the greater preload caused by a large, blunt needle (Weber-Fechner law).[15] The fibrous framework of the orbit, which attaches to the eye and the optic nerve, does not allow the vital structures to move out the way as has been proposed. The true situation in the orbit, according to Grizzard, is analogous to a full pickle jar, not a nearly empty one! He further states that "the most dangerous situation for a block is an ophthalmologist or anesthesiologist with a long, blunt needle who thinks ocular penetration and optic nerve damage are impossible."

Peribulbar anesthesia has been used since the late 1960's, according to C.P. Wilkinson, MD (written communication January 1988). It was formally described in March of 1986 by Davis and Mandel.[20] Their technique involves the use of multiple injection sites inferiorly and superiorly in a staged procedure. The technique does not incorporate a separate lid block. Cataract surgery utilizing a retrobulbar anesthetic without a separate seventh nerve block was first described by Gills and Loyd in 1983.[21] They described a modified retrobulbar injection through a transconjunctival approach using 2 to 3 cc of 0.75% bupivacaine posteriorly and 1 cc below the skin approximately 5 mm from the lateral canthus followed by mechanical orbital pressure for 60 minutes prior to surgery. In 1987 Kimbrough, et al presented their experience with a modification of the Gill's technique.[22] The technique as described is as follows: A retrobulbar needle (length unspecified) is passed through the lower lid at the junction of the lateral and middle third of the lower lid just above the inferior orbital margin. The needle is advanced approximately 1 1/4 inches. After aspiration, 3 to 4 cc of 0.75% marcaine is injected. As the needle is withdrawn, an additional 2 to 3 cc is injected. When the needle is in the subcutaneous tissue of the lid, pressure is applied with a finger medial to the needle while injecting an additional 4 to 5 cc of marcaine. This is followed by mechanical orbital pressure for 20 minutes prior to surgery.

Bloomberg and Wang[23,24] described modified versions of the peribulbar technique originally described by Davis and Mandel[20] although their technique also utilized two injection sites. Weiss and Deichman[25] performed a prospective, randomized, masked study of 79 consecutive cataract extractions with intraocular lens implantation comparing one injection site retrobulbar anesthesia and one injection site peribulbar anesthesia. In all cases the volume of anesthetic agent (50:50 mixture of 2% lidocaine hydrochloride and 0.75% bupivacaine hydrochloride) was 5 cc. They were unable to detect any significant difference in the two methods when evaluating globe anesthesia and akinesia and lid akinesia. They did note a higher incidence of conjunctival chemosis with peribulbar anesthesia. Supplemental anesthesia was required in 8(21%) of 39 patients in the retrobulbar group and 11(28%) of 39 patients in the peribulbar group. It was their conclusion that utilizing a single injection site combined with a low volume of anesthetic agent gave equivalent combined anesthesia and akinesia when compared to retrobulbar anesthesia and may be safer due to avoiding the muscle cone.

In January of 1988, we undertook a prospective, randomized double blinded study comparing retrobulbar and peribulbar anesthesia.[26] We compared 50 patient eyes undergoing standard retrobulbar anesthesia combined with O'Brien lid block with 50 patient eyes undergoing one injection site peribulbar anesthesia. The one injection site peribulbar block was performed utilizing a 26-gauge, 7/8 inch (22 mm), sharp needle place infraorbitally, one finger width medial to the lateral canthus. The needle was inserted through the inferior orbital septum until the hub of the needle was flush with the skin. Five cc of 50:50 mixture of 2% xylocaine and 0.75% bupivacaine with 5 units of Wydase per cc was injected slowly. The needle was then withdrawn to the subcutaneous space where an additional 5 cc of anesthetic was injected forming a skin wheal. Mechanical orbital pressure was then applied for 30 minutes prior to cataract surgery. We were unable to demonstrate a statistical difference between the two methods when evaluating lid akinesia, globe akinesia or globe anesthesia. Four of 50 patients in the retrobulbar group required reinjection (8%), while six of 50 patients in the peribulbar group (12%) received additional anesthesia.

Currently we use the above mentioned technique exclusively, on all patients undergoing procedures requiring local anesthesia. Prior to peribulbar injection the patient is given 0.5 to 2.0 mg of Versed (midazolam HC1) IV followed in five minutes by 100 to 120 mg of Surital (thiamylal sodium) (180–200 mg if Versed is not used). The patient is constantly monitored during this time by a certified registered nurse anesthetist. The peribulbar injection is performed approximately one to three minutes following administration of the Surital. The Patient is unconscious for approximately three to five minutes. A Honan balloon is applied immediately after the injection for approximately 30 minutes prior to surgery. If additional globe akinesia is necessary, a retrobulbar injection of 1 to 2 cc of a 50:50 mixture of 2% xylocaine and 0.75% marcaine is administered through a 25-gauge 1 1/4 inch needle. This is usually performed in the operating room just prior to prepping the patient. Supplemental sedation is unnecessary since the previous peribulbar anesthetic has anesthetized the skin and the orbital structures through which the needle passes.

Local anesthesia, delivered by means of a shorter needle out of the muscle cone, should theoretically eliminate the complications of CNS side effects from intradural injection and optic nerve injury. As might be anticipated, the risk of globe perforation has not been eliminated.[27] It is interesting that the perforation in the case described in this communication occurred at the site of the supranasal injection. According to a letter from W.S. Grizzard, MD in January 1990, eight cases of double perforating injuries following peribulbar anesthesia have been referred to his group. In each case, anesthesia was performed by an anesthesiologist. He did not indicate if multiple injections sites were utilized. Perhaps limiting the technique to one injection site may reduce further the possibility of occurrence of this complication.

Historically, one of the criticisms of peribulbar anesthesia has been its inability to provide adequate anesthesia for intraocular surgery. Also, at least 20 minutes of orbital pressure is required for diffusion of the anesthetic agent. These are definite disadvantages for vitreoretinal surgery. However, the routine use of a mechanical pressure device such as a Honan balloon or Super Pinkie prior to cataract surgery negates the latter disadvantage. The recent studies described herein leads one to believe adequate ocular anesthesia is obtainable by the periocular method. Vitreoretinal surgeons will most certainly continue to utilize retrobulbar anesthesia for manipulation of deeper ocular structures.

Summary

Complications of retrobulbar anesthesia include retrobulbar hemorrhage, respiratory depression, CNS side effects from intradural or subarachnoid injection, optic nerve contusion and atrophy, and perforation of the globe. One injection site peribulbar anesthesia using a 7/8 inch needle has been shown to be equal in efficacy to retrobulbar anesthesia with supplemental seventh nerve anesthesia for lid and globe akinesia and globe anesthesia. Advantages of peribulbar anesthesia should eliminate the complications of CNS side effects and optic nerve injury. Sharp needles are no more likely to cause complications than blunt needles. Finally, regardless of the technique utilized for ocular anesthesia, attention to detail is necessary to prevent complications.

References

1. Knapp H. On cocaine and its use in ophthalmic and general surgery. Arch of Ophthalmol 1884;13:402–08.
2. Atkinson WS. Local anesthesia in ophthalmology. Am J of Ophthal 1948;31:1607–18.
3. Koornneef L. Spatial aspects of orbital muscolo-fibrous tissue in man. Swets & Zeitlinger, Amsterdam.
4. Unsold R, Stanley JA, DeGroot J. The CT-topography of retrobulbar anesthesia. Albrecht vonGraefes Arch Klin Exp Ophthalmol, 217:137–42.
5. Castren JA, Tammisto T. A clinical evaluation of a new local anesthetic (marcaine-adrenalin) in ocular surgery. Acta Ophthalmol 1966;44:837–42.
6. Carolan, JA, Cerasol JR and Houle TV. Bupivacaine in retrobulbar anesthesia. Annals of Ophthal 1974;6:843–47.
7. Ellis PP. Retrobulbar injections. Surv Ophthalmol 1974;18:425–30.
8. Klein ML, Jampol LM, Condon PL, et al. Central retinal artery occlusion without retrobulbar hemorrhage after retrobulbar anesthesia. Am J Ophthalmol 1982;93:573–77.
9. Sullivan KL, Brown GC, Forman AR, et al. Retrobulbar anesthesia and retinal vascular obstruction. Ophthalmology 1983; 90:373–77.

10. Smith JL. Retrobulbar marcaine can cause respiratory arrest. J Clin Neuro-Ophthalmol 1982;1:171–2.

11. Chang JL, Gonzalez-Abola E, Larson CE, Lobes L. Brain stem anesthesia following retrobulbar block. Anesthesiology 1984;61:789–90.

12. Van Newkirk M. Personal communication, 1983.

13. Wittpenn JR, Rapoza P, Sternberg P, Kawashima L, Saklad J, Patz A. Respiratory arrest following retrobulbar anesthesia. Ophthalmol 1986:93:867–70.

14. Smith JL. Retrobulbar bupivacaine can cause respiratory arrest. Editorial Ann Ophthalmol 1982;14:1005–6.

15. Drysdale DB. Experimental subdural retrobulbar injection of anesthetic. Ann Ophthalmol 16;716–18.

16. Antoszyk AN, Buckley EG. Contralateral decreased visual acuity and extraocular muscle palsies following retrobulbar anesthesia. Ophthalmology 93:462–65.

17. Friedbert HL, Kline OR. Contralateral amaurosis after retrobulbar injection. Am J Ophthalmol 101:668–90.

18. Javitt JC, Addiego R, Friedberg HL, Libonati MM, Leahy JJ. Brain stem anesthesia after retrobulbar block. Ophthalmology 94:718–24.

19. Drysdale DB. Experimental subdural retrobulbar injection of anesthetic. Ann Ophthalmol 16:716–18.

20. Davis DB, Mandel MR. Posterior peribulbar anesthesia: An alternative to retrobulbar anesthesia. J Cataract Refract Surg 1986;12:182–84.

21. Gills JP, Loyd TL. A technique of retrobulbar block with paralysis of orbicularis oculi. Am Intraocular Implant Soc 1983;9:339–40.

22. Kimbrough RL, Stewart RH, Okereke PC. A modified Gill's block and its effectiveness for lid muscle akinesia. Ophthalmic Surg 18:14–17.

23. Bloomberg LB. Administration of peribulbar anesthesia. J of Cataract Refract Surg 1986;12:677–79.

24. Wang HS. Peribulbar anesthesia for ophthalmic procedures. J Cataract Refract Surg 1988;14:441–43.

25. Weiss JL, Deichman CB. A comparison of retrobulbar and peribulbar anesthesia for cataract surgery. Arch Ophthalmol 1989;107:96–98.

26. Whitsett JC, Balyeat HD, McClure B. Comparison of one-injection site peribulbar anesthesia and retrobulbar anesthesia. J Cataract Refract Surg. 1990;16:243–245.

27. Kimble JA, Morris RE, Witherspoon CD, et al. Globe perforation from peribulbar injection. Arch Ophthalmol 1987;105:749.

Chapter 2

CURRENT SURGICAL TECHNIQUES OF THE CAPSULE

Howard V. Gimbel, MD

The sixties heralded a new era in cataract surgery especially with the development of phacoemulsification by Dr. Charles Kelman. Ever since, small incision cataract surgery has been in continuous development. With the refinement of extracapsular and endocapsular cataract extraction techniques, the preference for in-the-bag posterior chamber intraocular lenses (PC-IOLs), and the evolution in soft or foldable IOL designs, came the demand for advancement in anterior capsulotomy/capsulectomy techniques.

Traditional capsulotomy/capsulectomy openings ranged from capsule forceps openings in the anterior capsule to slit-like ones.[1] More controlled V-shaped or small circular capsulectomies done by multiple tears were also performed.[2] To date there are various established techniques for opening. The capsulectomies are performed variously by air or irrigating cystotomes, by bent needles, by capsule scissors and forceps. The 1987 ASCRS Practice Styles Preference Survey reported that 89% of ophthalmologists used cystotome multiple punctures for anterior capsulectomy, 4% used YAG laser, 3% used a cystotome continuous tear, 3% used scissors, and 2% used some other anterior capsulotomy technique.[9] This compared to a 1989 Ocular Surgery News Anterior Capsulotomy Preference Survey of 500 ophthalmologists which reported 74% in favor of can-opener, 22% preferred capsulorhexis, and 2% each did Christmas-tree and intercapsular slits (OSN supplement, Nov. 15/89, p. 5). There appears to be a growing consensus among anterior segment surgeons in their preference for continuous circular capsulorhexis.

The well recognized merits of in-the-bag intraocular lens implantation are focusing the attention of surgeons on techniques that open the capsule, remove the cataract and still maintain an intact capsular bag in which to implant and center an IOL. The growing preference for Continuous Circular Capsulorhexis (CCC) as co-developed by the author and Dr. Thomas Neuhann is a reflection on the technique's multiple advantages. These advantages over current capsulotomies/capsulectomies have been discussed previously.[4,6]

Precise CCC that preserves the architecture of the capsular bag is proving to be one of the most important advancements in small incision cataract and lens implantation surgery. The revolutionary concept of circular capsular openings by continuous tear as achieved by CCC has contributed significantly to the safety and efficacy of cataract extraction and IOL implantation. Intraoperative and post-operative merits of CCC have been well documented.[4,6] Two-Staged Capsulorhexis as developed by the author in 1988 extends the possibilities of using CCC in difficult or challenging cases.[6] The principles of a continuous curvilinear or circular tear can be surgically applied to the posterior capsule as well. Posterior Continuous Circular (PCCC) is a technique developed by the author that builds on the principles of CCC and is a technique used for managing certain posterior capsule (PC) tears or for making primary posterior capsule openings.[5] All continuous tear capsulorhexis surgical techniques of the lens capsule enhance visual rehabilitation and extend the chances of safe and secure in-the-bag IOL placement because they maintain the integrity of the capsular bag and preserve the natural stability of the anterior/posterior segment.

The main virtue of the CCC technique is that it allows for every possible size, shape and location of capsular openings. The resultant anterior capsule rim is resilient and free of capsule flaps or tags and thereby resistant to tearing, even when stretched during lens material removal or intraocular lens implantation. The smooth continuously torn circular opening meets all the demands of advanced small incision cataract and lens implant surgery. Without it as a complementary procedure, other developments such as hydrodissection, endocapsular, intercapsular, small incision extracapsular, and endolenticular phacoemulsification, in-the-bag placement of soft IOL's, and lens implantation in children may not have realized their full potential. Most recently CCC is proving to be crucial for proper and lasting centration of multifocal IOL's.

The development of CCC has been described in the literature.[4] I initiate CCC by making a single puncture in the centre of the capsule with the irrigating cystotome. The tear is then guided radially out to the periphery at 3 o'clock where it is turned and continued around the capsule counterclockwise (Figures 2-1 and 2-2). The progressing tear is completed at the point where the initial radial tear had been turned circumferentially (Figures 2-3a and 2-3b). If the completion occurs more centrally onto the radial tear, the integrity of the edge is still maintained because of the obtuse angle at the junction where the tears meet.

These are the advantages to starting with the first puncture centrally and then guiding the continuous tear circumferentially. Other authors suggest starting the tear near or in the diameter of the tear. A central puncture reduces the tendency for inadvertent extension of the tear to the equator of the capsule, and makes it easier to re-engage the final part of the tear with its beginning. The best control of the progressing tear is achieved by grasping the developing capsular flap with the desired instrument close to where the capsule is tearing at the time. Resolving tangential vector forces allow for the direction of the tear to be controlled

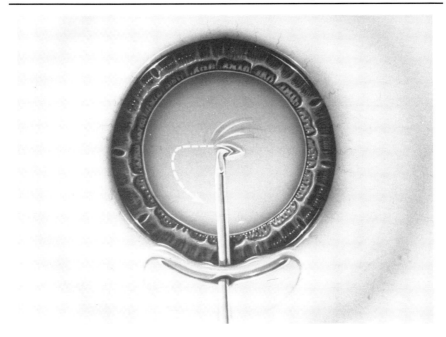

Figure 2-1: CCC is initiated by making a single puncture in the centre of the capsule and the tear is then guided radially to the periphery at 3 o'clock.

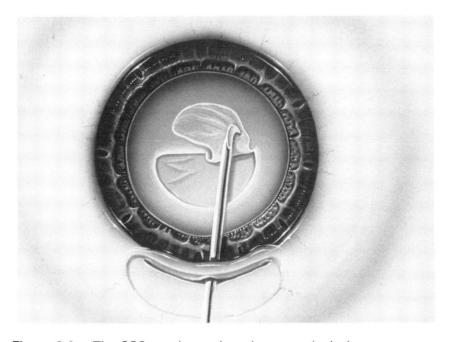

Figure 2-2: The CCC tear is continued counterclockwise.

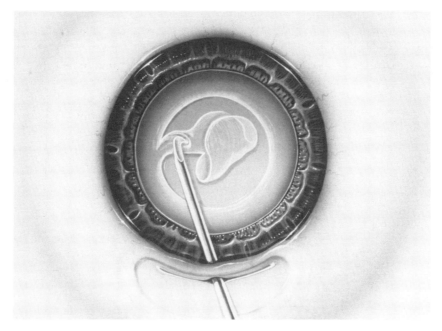

Figure 2-3a: CCC progressing tear is completed at point where initial radial tear had been turned.

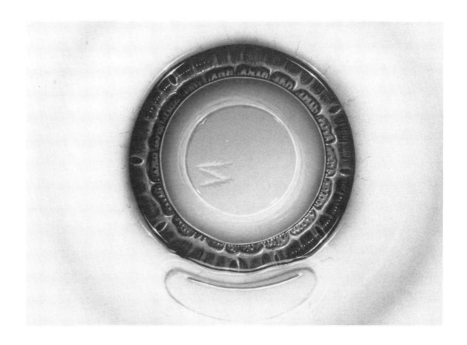

by the instrument's position and direction of force. Placing the tip of the instrument slightly ahead of the advancing tear will direct it more peripherally or centrifugally. Placing it slightly behind the tear will direct it centripetally. The tear may progress more smoothly and faster when the instrument is placed closer to the center of the radius, but less control can be maintained. When performing CCC on young people, it is necessary to pronouncedly direct the tear in a more central direction than usual since it tends to direct itself more peripherally. This tendency is greatest with increased convexity of the anterior surface of the capsule.

Making the original puncture centrally inside the proposed circle of the tear also reduces stress on the delicate zonules and enables the surgeon to choose the desired diameter of the capsulorhexis in small pupil cases or after decompression of the lens in intumescent cases.

There are rare cases where no form of CCC may be achieved. These include capsules that are heavily fibrosed and shrunken as in some congenital and traumatic cataracts. In these cases the anterior capsule needs to be cut with capsule scissors. In a partially fibrosed anterior capsule an opening may be achieved by combining CCC in the normal part of the capsule with scissor cuts of the fibrotic portions.

There are now almost as many ways of performing CCC as there are surgeons performing it. No single method is necessarily better than the other. Cystotomes, bent needles and forceps can all be used effectively. Anterior chamber pressure is maintained by air, BSS irrigation or by viscoelastic agents. Tear patterns may vary and progress clockwise or counterclockwise.

In my practice, CCC is completed without the use of viscoelastic in over 90% of cases. The viscoelastic Healon (R) is used in cases with positive vitreous or lens pressure, to break posterior synechiae, to enhance visualization of the capsule in small pupils, in cases with shallow anterior chambers, in pediatric cases, and is used, if a capsule forcep is used, to control and redirect a capsulorhexis that inadvertently begins to turn out too far radially into the periphery and zonules. Healon is used almost routinely in the second stage of Two-Staged Capsulorhexis technique and is always required in Posterior Continuous Circular Capsulorhexis.

Two-Staged Capsulorhexis extends the possibilities of achieving CCC in challenging and complicated cases. This technique is employed 1) for corneal endothelial protection in inter and endocapsular cataract extraction: 2) when the original capsulectomy is made purposefully small for safety reasons or can-opener like because of poor visualization in mature, opaque intumescent cataracts: 3) in small pupil cases where an originally small CCC requires subsequent conversion to a larger capsulectomy: 4) when the original capsulectomy is made inadvertently small: 5) conversion of small traumatic anterior capsule openings to CCC.[6]

In these situations, the initial small anterior capsule opening is converted to the desired diameter for IOL placement. The conversion is achieved by using both capsule scissors and the forceps. The original small capsulectomy may be large enough to admit the phaco probe for nucleus removal but too small for thorough removal of cortical material and placement of the IOL. After the lens nucleus is removed, the small initial opening is converted to a larger one of the desired diameter while still maintaining the continuous tear edge.

There is a growing consensus that the capsule opening should be kept relatively small, about 1.5 mm smaller than the selected IOL, since a large opening provides less support for the IOL and introduces additional risks for the tears to extend out to the equator as the tear crosses anterior zonule attachments. Whether the CCC is made purposefully or inadvertently small, it is amenable for enlargement to the desired diameter by a technique that I called Two-Staged Capsulorhexis.

Small pupil cases are still candidates for CCC and phacoemulsification.[3] If the pupil is small, the capsulectomy needs to be small for better visualization of the capsular edge during capsulorhexis and for certification of complete in-the-bag IOL placement. It is useful to use a second instrument through a side paracentesis in order to hold the pupillary margin aside. In performing CCC on a small pupil, the motion of tearing the capsule centripetally moves the side of the lens into view, making it possible to actually see and tear an opening that is larger than the pupil diameter. By gently stretching the opening into an elliptical shape, a 6.0 mm PMMA lens or a foldable lens may pass through a 4.0 mm capsular opening.

If the first capsulectomy is too small for admittance of an IOL, a second capsulectomy is started with a tangential snip on one side of the opening with capsule scissors (Figure 2-4). This is most safely accomplished with a viscoelastic agent such as Healon in the anterior chamber and in the

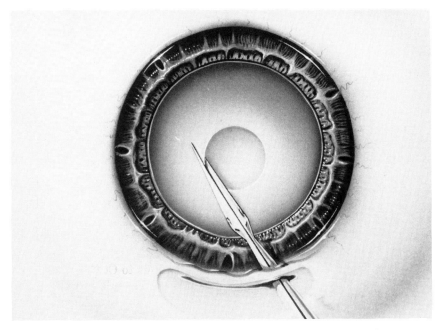

Figure 2-4:   Two-Staged CCC is started with a tangential snip on one side of the opening with capsule scissors.

lens capsule. It is crucial to prevent the side of the opening from folding over or under at the scissor tip so as to prevent a V cut. Such a cut would destroy the integrity of the continuous tear.

Once the tangential cut is successfully achieved, the second continuous tear is then extended using Kelman-McPherson or Kraff-Utrata forceps to complete a larger circle which is centered on the pupil and is of the desired diameter (Figure 2-5). The forceps are used to enlarge the original capsulectomy by removing a strip or ribbon of additional capsule (Figure 2-6). As with the original capsulectomy, the forces applied in making this tear have to be varied in order to guide the continuous tear in the desired direction (Figure 2-7).

This technique of using forceps to modify the original capsulectomy by removing additional capsule is also used in blunting or turning back short anterior capsule tears at the anterior capsule rim.[7]

In dense or intumescent cataracts where there is little or no red reflex, visualization of the anterior capsule is difficult. Increasing the magnification intensity of the operating microscope, dimming the operating room lights, and instilling viscoelastic substances into the anterior chamber or between the capsule and the cortex can prove helpful. If a slit-like or can-opener capsulectomy is all that can be achieved because of poor visualization, it can be converted into a CCC by Two-Staged Capsulorhexis as described.

The principles of surgical techniques of the anterior capsule can be extended to the posterior capsule. Posterior Circular Capsulorhexis (PCCC) employs the principles of CCC and is used to advantage when a small linear or triangular tear inadvertently occurs in the posterior capsule.[5]

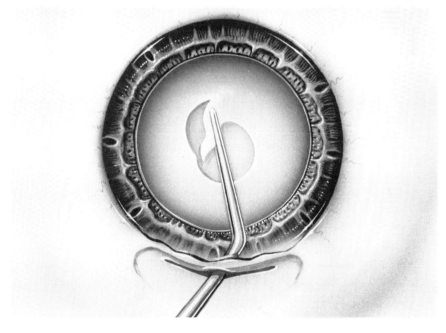

Figure 2-5: Two-Staged CCC is performed using forceps.

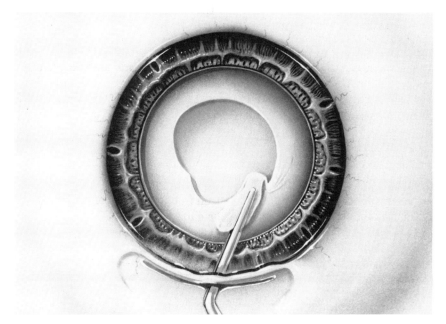

Figure 2-6:   Desired amount of additional capsule is removed.

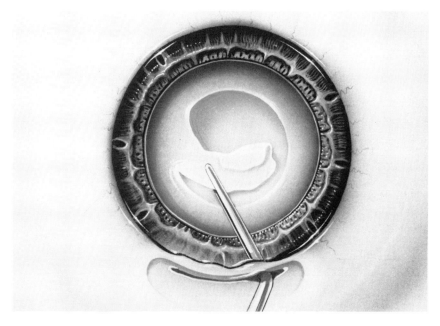

Figure 2-7:   Two-Staged CCC being completed.

In cases where such tears occur without extension too far toward the equator of the capsule, it is advantageous to accomplish a PCCC just as one does a CCC. Posterior capsule tears at the equator, or with extensions to the equator, are not amenable to PCCC. PCCC can also be used in the making of primary posterior capsulectomies.[1,10] I currently do not perform primary capsulectomies and vitrectomies in pediatric cataract and IOL cases, although I have not used IOL's in children under the age of 2.5 years.[8]

In converting an inadvertent tear by PCCC, one point of the advancing tear in the posterior capsule is extended and completed into a circle that encompasses the extent of the tear and is blended from the periphery (Figure 2-8). Alternatively one or both ends of a linear tear may be rounded or blunted. The best control of the progressing tear in the posterior capsule is achieved using the elongated Kelman-McPherson or Kraff-Utrata forceps, grasping the capsule flap near one point of tearing and turning the tear in the desired direction (Figure 2-9).[5] My current practice is to convert all PC tears that are amenable by PCCC.

The PCCC is kept as small as possible so as to preserve the maximum support of the posterior capsule. This technique is performed in order to avoid an anticipated extension of the inadvertent linear or triangular tear during such maneuvers as a required vitrectomy or lens placement. Similarly if a primary posterior capsulectomy is required to preserve a clear visual axis in infants and children, it may be done by using PCCC to avoid tears that extend to the equator of the capsule.[1,10] PCCC can also be employed for the removal of a thickened fibrotic posterior capsule

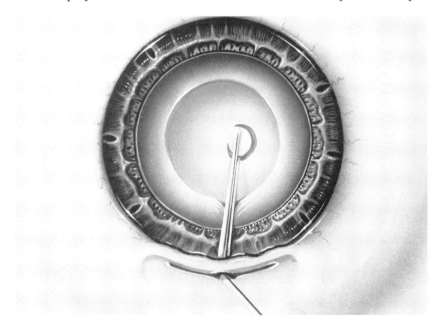

Figure 2-8: PCCC is performed using forceps to grasp one point of the advancing tear.

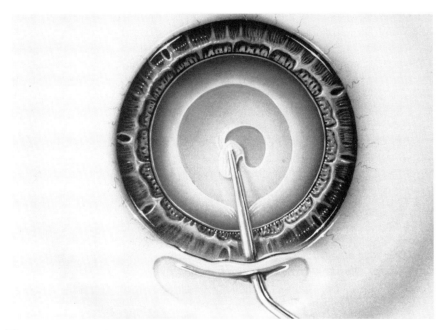

Figure 2-9: PCCC-Forceps directing tear in desired direction.

plaque. In these cases, the PCCC is made as a controlled circle that encompasses the central opacity and results in a posterior capsule opening that resists extension to the equator from the capsule contracture that occurs in the months following surgery with possible posterior dislocation of the IOL (Figure 2-10). The initial puncture has to be outside the circumference of the plaque and close to the desired diameter of the posterior capsulectomy. This posterior capsular opening can be made after the IOL is implanted in the bag. Using a viscoelastic agent, the IOL is nudged eccentrically and a barbed needle on a syringe of viscoelastic is slipped under the IOL.[5]

The multiple advantages of performing CCC highlight the anterior segment surgeon's concern for security of capsular bag integrity by prevention of unwarranted radial tears or tags, in the-bag IOL placement, and IOL centration and verification.[4,6] In phacoemulsification cataract extraction cases with lens implantation, early suspicion and/or detection of anterior or posterior capsule tears can convert a potentially less than acceptable post-operative result into an acceptable or perfect one.

From our studies it has been our experience that there are risks of anterior and posterior capsule tears at every stage of cataract extraction with IOL placement.[5,7] In a two month series, 6 or 0.88% anterior capsule tears and 4 or 0.58% posterior capsule tears occurred in a total of 682 consecutive phacoemulsification cases operated between September 1 and October 31, 1989.[7] In a two year study 1987–89 for PC tears, 36 or 0.5% PC breaks occurred in 7,169 phacoemulsification cataract cases.[5] To date, to the best of our knowledge, no other phacoemulsification series ana-

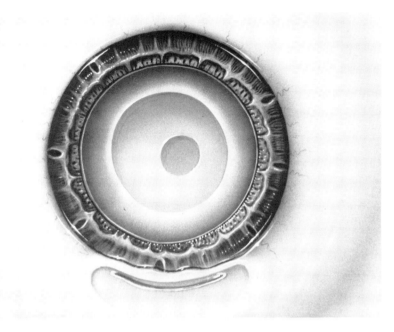

Figure 2-10:   Completed PCCC.

lyzing capsule defects has been published. We refer to our experience that isolated AC or PC tears, or AC tear extensions into the posterior capsule may occur at any time during surgery from anterior capsulorhexis to lens implantation, and that AC tears extending to the posterior capsule lead to the greatest intra/post-operative complications.[5]

Late complications can often be avoided when earlier ones, especially AC tears, are managed. AC tears extending from the anterior capsulectomy are best prevented by accomplishing a smooth, continuous, circular opening as achieved with CCC. No irregular flaps or tags are left to interfere with surgery. There is no need to create a superior flap for access of cortical clean-up at the 12 o'clock position as this superior cortex is easily removed using a bent cannula through the paracentesis at the horizontal limbus or through the main incision using a Binkhorst cannula.

While generally very beneficial, there is one risk peculiar to CCC.[4] The edge of the capsulorhexis may contract a few months post-operatively with the propensity to purse-string contracture. This contracture rarely leads to any significant degree of IOL decentration but with very weak zonules, the contracture can progress to produce a central opacity. This can be stopped by making multiple cuts in the ring using the Nd:Yag laser. James A. Davison recently discussed what he believes to be the first reported complication of capsulorhexis: distention of the capsular bag after phaco and PC-IOL implantation.[11] We have not witnessed this particular complication possibly because we evacuate Healon from behind the IOL as well as from the anterior chamber.

The benefits of CCC make it increasingly the technique of choice for all cataract surgeons. It can be performed in several ways, and it has been proven to be consistently reproducible by experienced surgeons. Because of the cellophane-like qualities of the anterior capsule, some ophthalmologists have learned CCC by practicing on cellophane wrap stretched over a glass.[12] For surgeons doing extracapsular surgery, since a 4.5 mm capsulorhexis is optimum, one can practice CCC and then go outside of it to do the routine can-opener capsulectomy, so each case can be practice. We believe that the technique can be learned and performed consistently by every experienced cataract surgeon.

CONCLUSION

It has been our experience that continuous tear capsulorhexis techniques of the lens capsule decrease the potential of intraoperative radial tears of either the anterior or posterior capsule. Prevention of anterior capsule tears by achieving CCC or management of inadvertent short AC tears by partial Two-Staged Capsulorhexis optimizes capsular bag integrity. Extension of CCC principles to challenging or complicated cases by Two-Staged or Double Capsulorhexis, or prevention of the progression of inadvertent PC tears by PCCC also optimizes the maintenance of the capsular bag for IOL placement.

References

1. Dahan E: Lens Implantations in Microphthalmic Eyes of Infants. European Journal of Implant and Refractive Surgery, 1, 1989, 9–11.
2. Emery JM, Little JH: Phacoemulsification and aspiration of Cataracts, St. Louis, 1969, Mosby, 79–95.
3. Gimbel HV, Nesbitt JAA: Small pupil: An indication for phacoemulsification. Upcoming publication Canadian Journal of Ophthalmology.
4. Gimbel HV, Neuhann T: Development, advantages and methods of the Continuous Circular Capsulorhexis technique, Journal of Cataract and Refractive Surgery, 16, 1990, 31–37.
5. Gimbel HV: Posterior Capsule Tears Using Phacoemulsification: Causes, prevention and management. Upcoming publication March 1990 European Journal of Implant and Refractive Surgery.
6. Gimbel HV: Two Staged Capsulorhexis for Endocapsular Phacoemulsification. Upcoming publication Journal of Cataract and Refractive Surgery.
7. Gimbel HV: Continuous Circular, Two Staged, and Posterior Continuous Circular Capsulorhexis: Description and Analysis. Upcoming publication in Ophthalmic Practice.
8. Gimbel HV: Continuous Circular Capsulorhexis: The Key to Successful in-the-bag Posterior Implants in Children. Upcoming publication.

9. Leaming DV: Practice Styles and Preference of ASCRS Member 1987 Survey. Journal of Cataract and Refractive Surgery, 14, 1988, 552–559.

10. Parks MA: Posterior lens Capsulectomy during primary cataract surgery in Children. Ophthalmology 1983, 90:344–345.

11. Davison JA: Distention of the capsular bag after phaco and posterior chamber IOL implantation—a unique complication of capsulorhexis. Ocular Surgery News, 7(21):18.

12. Fine IH: Preferred techniques for single-stitch cataract/IOL surgery. Ocular Surgery News—Supplement, 7(22):6.

Chapter 3

EVIDENCE IN SUPPORT OF THE CONTINUOUS TEAR ANTERIOR CAPSULECTOMY (CAPSULORHEXIS TECHNIQUE)

David J. Apple, MD
Ehud I. Assia, MD
Daniel Wasserman, MD
Julie C. Tsai, MD
Victoria E. Castaneda, MD
Todd D. Gwin, MD
Sandra J. Brown, RN

Overview

In our laboratory we have demonstrated that the incidence of radial tears after "can-opener" anterior capsulectomy is very high (86%). The "pea-podding" effect and subsequent clinically significant complications such as decentration can occur after anterior capsular tears. We have demonstrated that the continuous circular capsulorhexis (CCC) procedure provides the most resistance to formation of irregular tears and their sequelae. We therefore recommend a transition towards this technique when feasible. The results of cataract surgery are already excellent and we predict even better overall long term results as more surgeon perform better and more exacting anterior capsulectomies.

Introduction

The most frequently performed forms of anterior capsulectomy with extra-capsular cataract extraction (ECCE) are the "can opener" technique, the linear (intercapsular or envelope) technique and the continuous circular capsulorhexis (CCC). The capsulorhexis technique and hydrodissection are now being popularized, particularly by phacoemulsification surgeons.

Does the smooth-edged circular anterior capsulectomy really provide an advantage? Does this technique really decrease the incidence of such complications as radial tears and secondary decentration, as opposed to the classic "can opener" technique?

With modern cataract surgery particular attention must be paid to achieving intraocular lens (IOL) centration and avoidance of decentration. This is primarily due to two factors: 1) an increased use of or return to smaller diameter optics (6mm or less) or aspherical optics (5 × 6mm) and 2) the increased and undoubtedly widespread future use of bifocal and/or multi-focal IOLs—that conceptually at least require good optic centration.

This article provides a summary of our experimental studies showing indeed that these reported advantages of the capsulorhexis capsulectomy are indeed real and therefore, merit increased use in the cataract surgeon's armamentarium.

The Evolution of the Anterior Capsulectomy

Ever since the return to ECCE as a popular and/or preferred surgical technique, which was greatly accelerated with the increased use of posterior chamber intraocular lenses (PC-IOLs) in the late 1970s, various types of anterior capsular openings have been used (Figure 3-1). These include the so-called Christmas tree type, the "can opener" type, the intercapsular technique, the "postage stamp" type, and more recently the continuous circular capsulorhexis (CCC).[1,2] The intercapsular technique, popularized in the late 1970's (reviewed in references 3 and 4) is basically a two-step capsulorhexis technique, an initial curvilinear incision or slit, followed by a completion of the anterior capsular opening following complete removal of lens substance and insertion of the IOL (Figure 3-2). Since intercapsular technique has been used since the late 1970s, the concept of capsulorhexis or tearing as a maneuver is not new. Note that the hoped-for results of both the classic intercapsular technique and the modern CCC are the same.

Anytime an anterior capsulectomy is performed in which a sharp or jagged edge or slit remains, there is a potential for radial tears towards the equator. Examples of this are shown in Figure 3-3, showing two experimental eyes with the intercapsular anterior capsulectomy. Each eye has a slit-like edge at the lateral margin of the anterior capsulectomy. In Figure 3-3A the opening has not extended. Figure 3-3B shows a high-power view of an eye where a radial tear has extended all the way to the equator after this technique. It follows that the main rationale for obtaining an anterior capsular opening that has a smooth, nonserrated edge is, by avoiding the formation of jagged or sharp edges, one will decrease the propensity for or incidence of radial tear formation. Therefore, justification of using the highly-touted CCC technique rests on answering two basic questions: 1) Are radial tears common with routine surgery such as with the "can opener" technique? and 2) If so, are they of clinical significance and could avoidance of tears therefore improve long-term results? These questions have been addressed in an excellent clinical

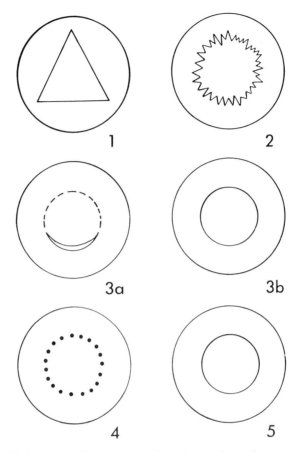

Figure 3-1: Schematic illustration showing selected types of anterior capsulectomy with ECCE.
1. "Christmas Tree" and 2. "can opener" techniques. Both of these are characterized by serrations or radial slits at the margins of the capsule.
3. Intercapsular or envelope technique, essentially a two-stage capsulorhexis. The horizontal, curvilinear slit (3a) is done initially, lens substance is removed and the IOL is inserted, and the opening is completed by tearing the remaining capsule (3b). The margins of the initial slit are generally pointed. They may therefore be susceptible to horizontal tears towards the equator.
4. Circular capsulectomy made by multiple punctures (postage-stamp type).
5. Continuous circular capsulorhexis (CCC), with smooth-edge tear. This is made in one step using either a bent needle or forceps; it may conceptually be considered to be an anterior capsulectomy formed by an infinite number of interconnected points.

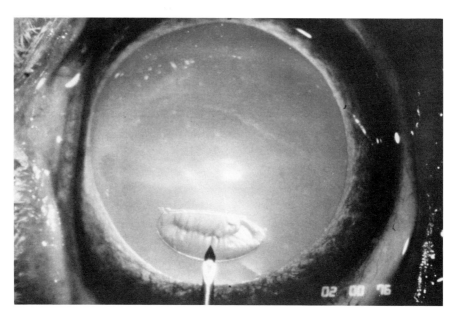

Figure 3-2: Examples of the intercapsular technique; operation performed on three experimental rabbit eyes.

Figure 3-2a: The initial horizontal or curvilinear slit.

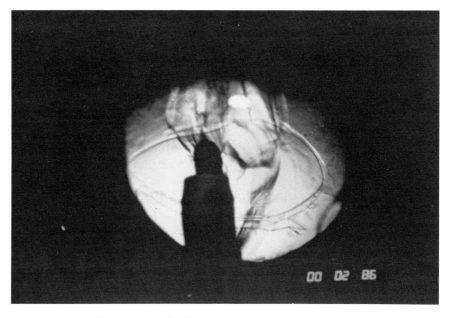

Figure 3-2b: The removal of lens substance by aspiration through the slit-like orifice.

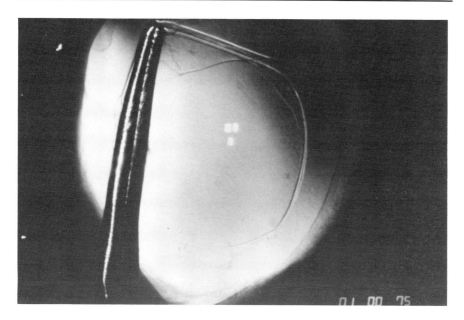

Figure 3-2c: The second stage of the capsulectomy, namely the tearing motion or capsulorhexis performed to complete the circular opening.

study[5] but to date have not been addressed using clinicopathological and experimental data.

Radial Tears: Incidence and Significance

A recent and important study by Wasserman and coauthors has shown that radial tears following the "can opener" technique are much more common than previously assumed.[6] In evaluating a series of 250 consecutive eyes obtained postmortem with PC-IOLs, one or more radial tears were noted in 86% of cases (Figures 3-3, 3-4, 3-5, and 3-6 and Table 3-1). This information has heretofore not been available from either clinical or pathological studies. This data is impossible to determine clinically in a systemic fashion because the mid- and far periphery of the lens, including the equatorial capsule are, of course, not visible to the surgeon. These are hidden behind the peripheral iris.

   This study[6] demonstrates conclusively that the incidence of capsular tears is indeed high.

   What then is the significance of such tears? It is well known from autopsy studies[3,7 and 8] that as many as 50 percent of PC-IOLs are implanted asymmetrically, one loop in the capsular bag and one loop out of or anterior to the capsular bag. It has generally been assumed that this is caused by surgical error in implantation. Our Miyake technique studies[9] in which

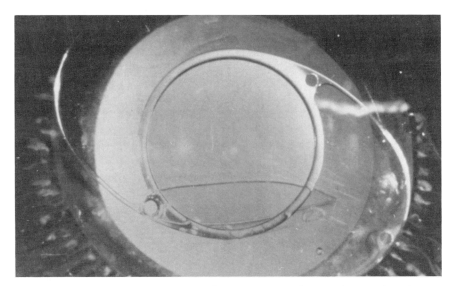

Figure 3-3a: Gross photograph from an experimental eye showing an implanted one piece modified C-loop IOL into the capsular bag after preparation of a horizontal slit anterior capsulectomy. Note that the horizontal edges of the tear are sharp and would be considered prone to extension, although it did not occur in this case.

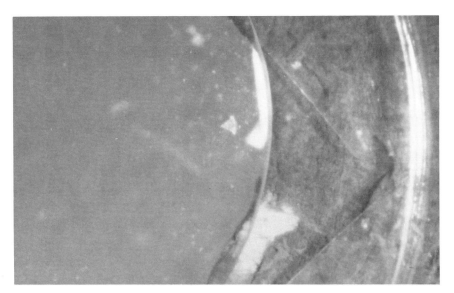

Figure 3-3b: Gross photograph from behind of a similar case showing the mid-periphery and periphery of the capsular bag after IOL implantation. Note that a larger radial extension of the intercapsular slit has occurred to the equator. Such an occurrence undoubtedly may set the stage for either intraoperative or postoperative dislocation of IOL loops, the so called pea-podding effect.

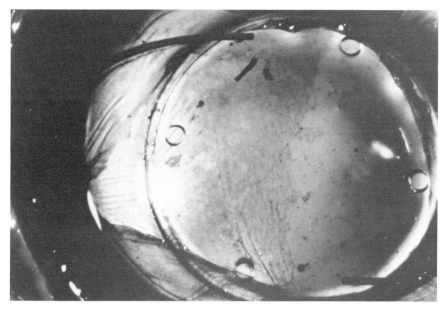

Figure 3-4:   Gross photograph from in front (cornea and iris removed) of a human eye obtained post-mortem in which a PC-IOL has been implanted. Using the periodic acid-Schiff (PAS) stain, a single radial tear (extending towards the left in this photograph) that had occurred clinically is visible.

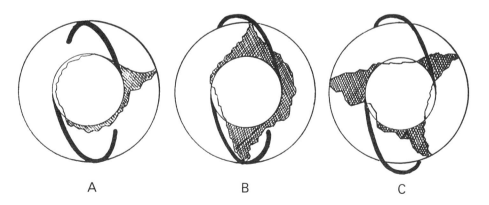

A   B   C

Figure 3-5:   Schematic illustration from the study by Wasserman and associates[6] showing examples of one, two, and three radial tears respectively. The stability and long term fixation of the loops, i.e. the avoidance of "pea-podding" or exit of loops from the capsular bag, partially depends on whether the loops (B & C)are situated in or near the sites of the tears or is/are situated away from the loop tips or lenses (A).

ANTERIOR CAPSULECTOMY
PERIPHERAL TEARS

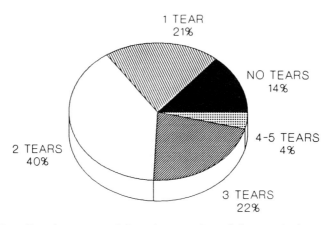

Figure 3-6: Graph summarizing the results of the study by Wasserman and coauthors,[6] showing tear-free anterior capsules in only 14% of a series of 250 consecutive autopsy eyes. In other words, following routine ECCE surgery with the "can opener" technique (as was generally the rule in the cases studied) one or more radial tears occurred in 86% of cases.

dynamic movements of the IOLs during implantation can be documented, suggest that asymmetric location of loops may be caused by the "pea-pod" effect. This is defined as an exit of an in-the-bag loop from the bag. This may, for example, occur during IOL dialing. The most common cause of this is either an insufficient, scanty anterior capsular flap or a radial

Table 3-1:

Number and morphology of anterior capsular tears in 250 post-mortem eyes. Note the one or more radial tears occur in 86% of cases, a surprising high figure.

TEAR(S)	NUMBER	PERCENT	
NO TEARS, REGULAR EDGES	22	9	} 14%
NO TEARS, IRREGULAR EDGES	12	5	
ONE TEAR	51	21	
TWO TEARS	100	40	} 86%
THREE TEARS	55	22	
FOUR-FIVE TEARS	10	4	

tear(s) such as discussed in this report. Therefore it follows that radial tears may indeed be deleterious in that they may increase the incidence of the complication of asymmetric fixation. This in turn increases the possibility of decentration and its sequelae.[10,11] Note also this correlates well with Figure 3-7 showing that in Wasserman's series,[6] the highest incidence of symmetric in-the-bag implantation was achieved in cases with only 0 to 1 tears.

The significance of radial tears as being potential contributing factors in or direct causes of decentration is further substantiated in studies of human eyes obtained postmortem with PC-IOLs,[10] in which as many as 8.1 percent of cases have loops that are situated in neither the capsular bag nor ciliary sulcus, but extend into the zonules or pars plana (Figure 3-8A and 3-8B). In at least some cases it can be presumed that these loops had exited ("pea-podded") from the capsular bag due to defects in the anterior capsule.

Efficacy and Rationale of the Continuous Circular Capsulorhexis (CCC) Technique

Assuming that anterior capsular radial tears are significant causes of decentration and therefore undesirable, does the continuous circular cap-

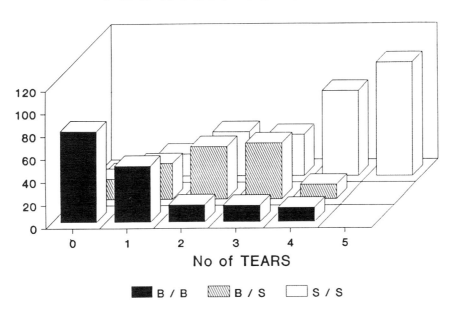

Figure 3-7: In Wasserman and associates series,[6] the frequency of symmetrical in-the-bag fixation of PC-IOL loops was directly related to the number of radial tears present. The eyes with zero or only one radial tear appeared to have the highest incidence of complete in the bag fixation.

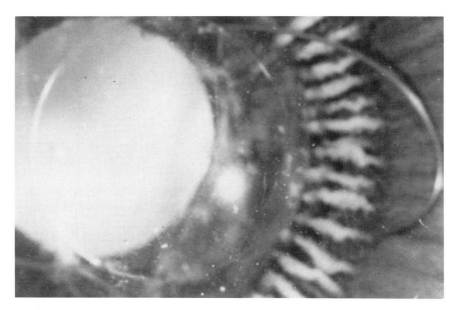

Figure 3-8: In approximately 8.1% of cases, zonular or pars plana fixation of loops occurs,[10] as opposed to the expected in-the-bag or ciliary sulcus fixation. No doubt in some of these cases the loops have extended posteriorly because of anterior capsular defects such as radial tears.

Figure 3-8a: Gross photograph from behind of a human eye obtained postmortem showing an example of a loop that was implanted neither in-the-bag or the ciliary sulcus, but rather has extended into the pars plana.

sulorhexis (CCC) technique indeed decrease the incidence of such tears? In order to assess this, elegant studies were performed by Assia and associates.[12,13] In the latter study forty human eyes obtained postmortem without previous surgical interventions, were divided into four groups of ten and anterior capsulectomies were performed as follows (Figure 3-1): Group 1: classic "can opener" technique; Group 2: intercapsular technique; Group 3: postage stamp (multiple fine punctures) technique; and Group 4: continuous circular capsulectomy (CCC) (capsulorhexis) technique. After completion of each capsulectomy, a controlled force was placed on the cut edge of the capsular margin in each case. As the force was gradually increased, by a controlled nuclear expression technique, ruptures or tears of the anterior capsule were documented. The results were conclusive (Figure 3-9). Without exception, the anterior capsular remnant in eyes with the CCC technique remained free of tears with the forces applied (Figures 3-9A and B). With the other three techniques, radial tears invariably occurred with equivalent or lesser force (Figures 3-9C and D). This represents the first controlled experimental study to dem-

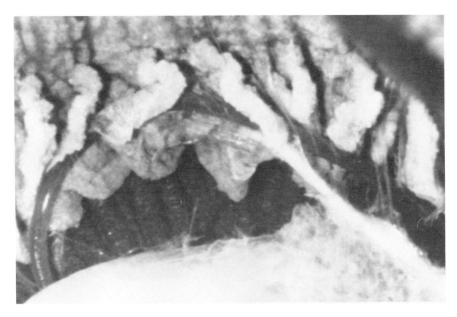

Figure 3-8b: Gross photograph from behind of another human eye obtained post-mortem with a PC-IOL prepared with the critical point drying technique (this photograph shows the loop extending onto the tips of the pars plicata).

onstrate the important point that the anterior capsular edge after capsulorhexis is highly resilient and resistant to tears as compared to the other techniques. This point has been widely touted and assumed clinically, and has been discussed in the tabloid literature, but until now has not been shown in an experimental fashion in the peer-reviewed literature.

Our studies have shown that, when any defect is present at the anterior capsular edge during the surgical procedure, the formation of a capsular tear such as illustrated in experimental studies (Figure 3-10) may occur at a low threshold of force and may be rapidly propagated. Figure 3-11 demonstrates the basic mechanism. A force may be applied to the edge of any membrane-like structure composed of interconnected molecules (for example, the anterior capsule). This force may be considered analogous to a force exerted on the capsule during lens substance removal or IOL implantation. If the edge is smooth, without any preformed defect, the forces are diffused and distributed along the edge (Figure 3-11A). If a pre-formed defect or slit (such as the serration of a "can opener" capsulectomy is present (Figure 3-11B), a force along the capsular edge would tend to separate the slit edges, thus widening the gap (Figure 3-11A and B). The major force would then be concentrated at an interior point C in Figure 3-11b, thus separating the molecules and propagating the tear. This principle may be demonstrated by considering a peanut bag (Figure 3-12). When no pre-cut slit at the edge of the bag is present, it may be

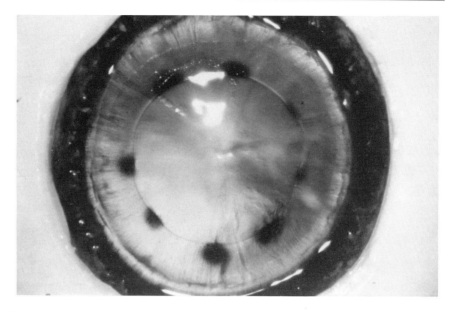

Figure 3-9:   Experimental comparison of anterior capsular tear resistance during two capsulectomy procedures. This study[13] demonstrates that the smooth-edge continuous tear capsulorhexis is most resistant to formation and extension of radial tears. All photographs are from the surgeon's view of human eyes obtained post-mortem. The cornea and iris were removed, the capsulectomy was performed, and the formation of tears during lens substance expression was evaluated.

Figure 3-9a: Continuous tear capsulorhexis, *before* nuclear expression, no radial tears.

difficult to open. When a pre-cut slit is present (Figure 3-12), bag opening is facilitated.

Clinicopathologic Observations on the Continuous Circular Capsulorhexis (CCC) Technique

The anterior capsular tear may be made using either a bent needle or cystotome, as originally advocated by Neuhann[1] and Gimbel,[2] or the forceps popularized by Peter Utrata of Columbus, Ohio. The details of the surgical technique are beyond the scope of this paper, but are reviewed by many authors.[1,2,14]

Figures 3-13A and B show laboratory examples of CCC. By achieving such a smooth edge as seen here, one minimizes the potential for radial tearing. The capsulorhexis is more amenable to the subsequent hydro-dissection technique which many surgeons recommend. The smooth edge of the capsule helps avoid tears as the aqueous fluid is injected through the capsulectomy.

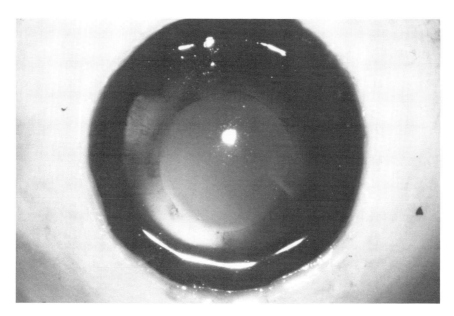

Figure 3-9b: Continuous tear capsulorhexis, *after* nuclear expression, with radial tear.

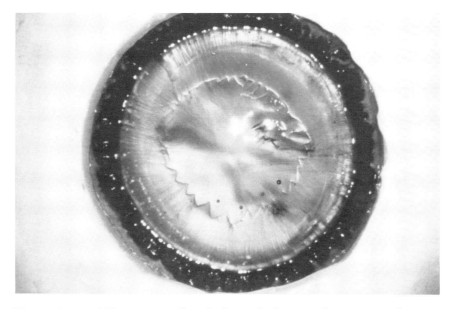

Figure 3-9c: "Can-opener" technique, *before* nuclear expression, with radial tear.

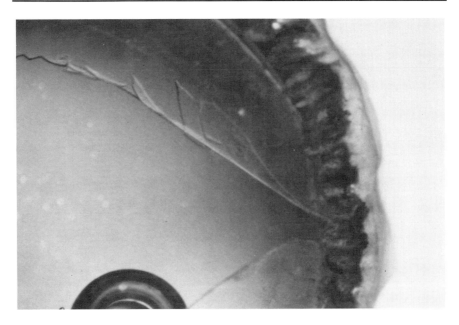

Figure 3-9d: "Can-opener" technique, *after* nuclear expression, with radial tear.

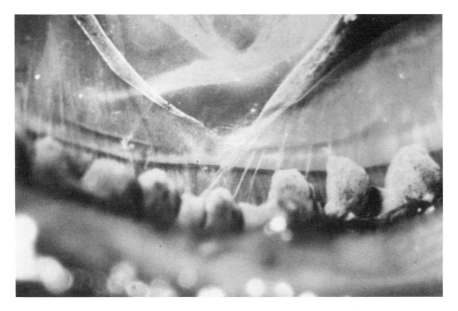

Figure 3-10:   Gross photograph from in front (surgeon's view, human autopsy globe, cornea and iris removed) an example of an experimental anterior capsular tear extending to the equator. Although it has been shown that these occur in 86% of cases,[6] Assia has shown that these rarely extend around the anterior equatorial capsule onto the posterior capsule.

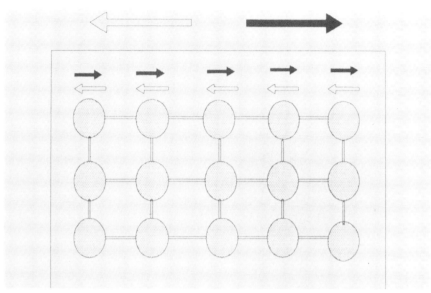

Figure 3-11a: Schematic illustration showing a membrane-like structure composed of interconnecting molecules. The edge of the membrane (above) is smooth. There is no disruption of the molecular structure as long as the edge of the membrane where the force is applied remains smooth and continuous, with no defect.

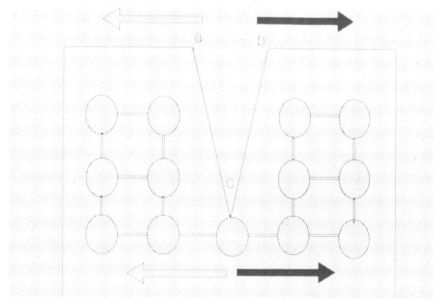

Figure 3-11b: If a defect, such as a serration or slit as illustrated here is present, the force applies to the edge of the membrane (above) causes a widening or gaping of the defect (a–b). The force then concentrates at (c), separating the molecules. This is the basic principle that explains the formation and extension of radial tears in cases where a preformed slit is present.

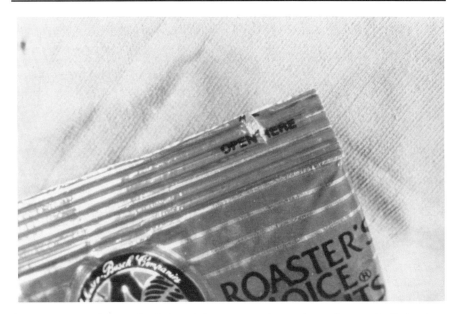

Figure 3-12:   The principle of the peanut bag. A preformed slit in the peanut bag as seen here facilitates the opening of the bag. A preformed tear of an anterior capsular edge facilitates radial tears.

The overwhelming majority, if not all, phacoemulsification surgeons are now using the capsulorhexis technique, since it is readily amenable to this technique and also facilitates the use of various small incision or foldable lenses. Figure 3-14A illustrates, in a laboratory model, the use of a very small diameter capsulorhexis (5–6mm)—often used with phacoemulsification. Note that a relatively large one-piece IOL was inserted through this relatively small anterior capsulectomy.

The technique has not generally been applied to standard ECCE procedures, but such use is possible. If capsulorhexis is to be used with nuclear expression in ECCE, the capsulectomy diameter in general must be greater (Figure 3-14B) and hydrodissection is essential. The anterior capsulectomy diameter with ECCE should generally be greater than 6.0mm, depending on the consistency of the cataractous lens.

Figure 3-15A illustrates in a laboratory model the technique of hydrodissection. This is a very useful technique to separate the various lamellae of the lens, including separation of capsule and cortex, cortex from nucleus, and various layers in between. Injection of an aqueous solution at various levels will separate individual lens lamellae, depending of course upon the consistency and hardness of the lens. With relatively soft lenses, it is actually possible to remove the entire lens substance with hydrodissection as illustrated in Figure 3-15B. Such extraction of the lens by hydrodissection is not recommended clinically. However, we have done this in our laboratory on numerous occasions.

We have that the CCC technique reasonably easy to perform in a consistent fashion, as have most surgeons who have adopted this proce-

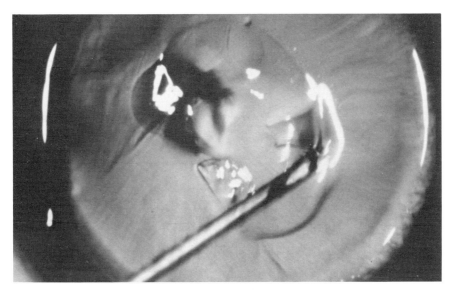

Figure 3-13:   Experimental creation of a continuous tear anterior capsulectomy (capsulorhexis) in a human eye obtained post-mortem, viewed from in front (surgeon's view) with the cornea and iris removed.

Figure 3-13a: Note in this case that the force that causes the capsular tear is generated by a pushing and pulling motion of a bent needle. The same effect can be achieved with a Utrata forceps.

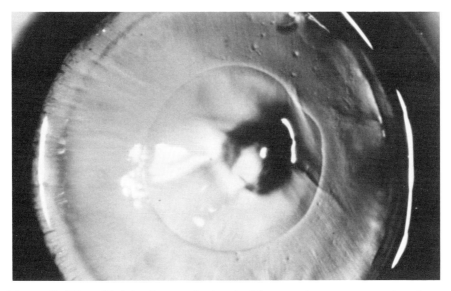

Figure 3-13b: Finished capsulorhexis. The continuous, smooth edge is resistant to radial tears and is also resistant to tearing and tag formation during the step of hydrodissection. During hydrodissection the internal pressure in the capsular bag and hence on the anterior capsule is slightly increased as the fluid is infused.

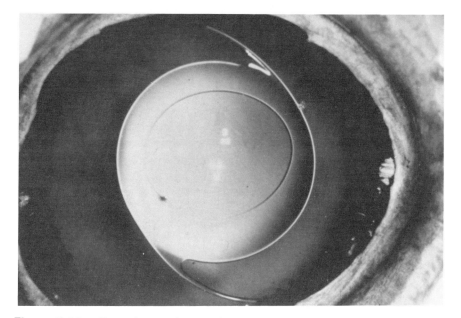

Figure 3-14:   Experimental capsulorhexis.

Figure 3-14a: Gross photograph of a porcine eye obtained post-mortem, after completion of capsulorhexis and insertion of a one piece PC-IOL. Note that the large lens (14.0 mm. tip to tip diameter) has been inserted through a very small (5.0 mm.) capsular orifice. Such small capsulectomies are frequently performed by phacoemulsification surgeons.

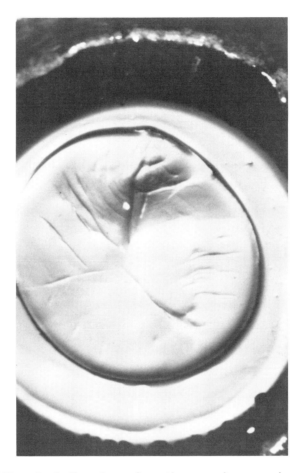

Figure 3-14b: A similar view of another porcine eye showing a much larger (6.5mm) capsulorhexis, viewed just prior to lens substance removal. Such relatively large openings are generally required for ECCE (non-phacoemulsification) procedures.

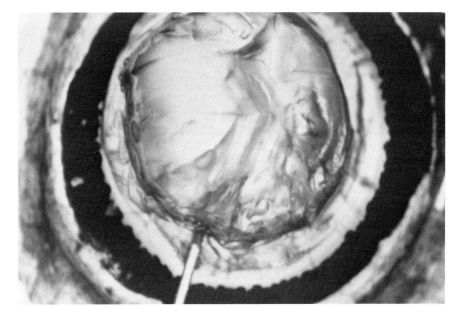

Figure 3-15:   Experimental hydrodissection in the lens of a porcine eye.

Figure 3-15a: Subcapsular injection of an aqueous or saline solution. As the fluid enters into the capsular bag the contents swell, and a pressure is exerted on the margins of the anterior capsular remnants, but no tears occur.

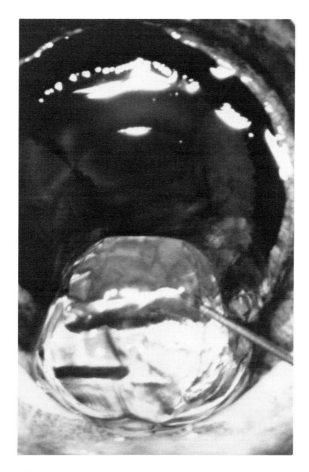

Figure 3-15b: The entire lens substance (cortex and nucleus) are expressed in its entirety through the capsulorhexis with no radial tear.

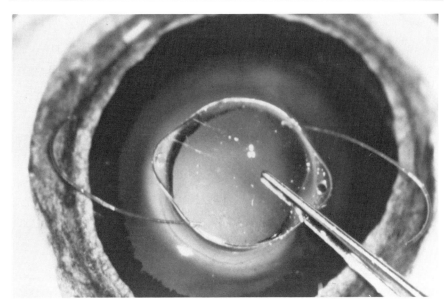

Figure 3-16: Experimental study demonstrating the principle of "pea-podding" (exit of IOL loops from the capsular bag) through an extending radial tear of the anterior capsule.

Figure 3-16a: Capsulorhexis and removal of lens substance have been performed and a 14 mm three piece modified J-loop IOL is ready for implantation.

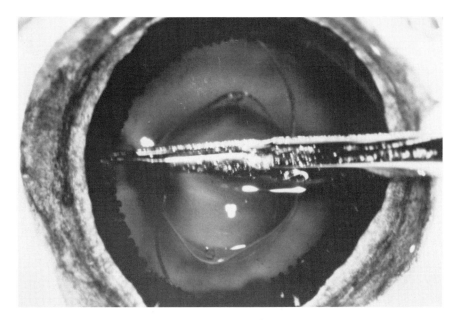

Figure 3-16b: After the IOL has been securely implanted with the loops oriented vertically, a planned experimental tear is performed (left), 90 degrees from the long axis of the IOL loops.

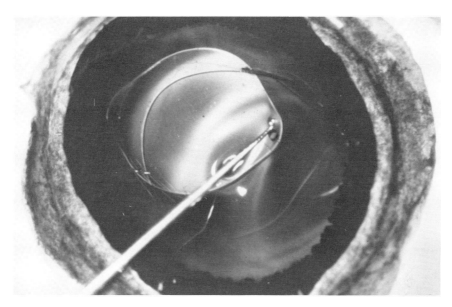

Figure 3-16c: As long as the IOL loops are situated perpendicular to the tear, in this case vertical, the lens remains securely fixated.

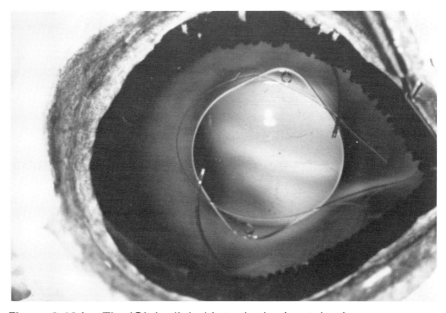

Figure 3-16d: The IOL is dialed into the horizontal axis.

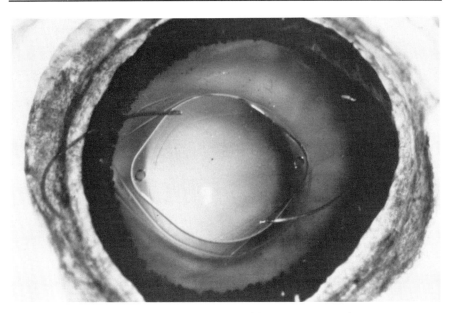

Figure 3-16e: As soon as the IOL loop is dialed into the site of the extended tear, it exits ("pea-pods") from the capsule via the rent and is situated anterior to the anterior capsule.

dure as a routine. Assuming that the technique is as easy, quick, and safe as the classic "can opener" technique, the rationale or bottom line for use of this procedure-prevention of tears, "pea-podding," and decentration—becomes clear. The major advantage of this technique can be illustrated from the laboratory perspective in Figures 3-16A–E. The sequence of events documented in Figures 3-16A–E, performed in our laboratory using a porcine eye, illustrates the precise mechanism of pea-podding through an anterior capsular defect. Note how a modified J-loop three-piece IOL (Figure 3-16A), implanted into the eye with a capsulorhexis, will exit from the capsular bag after the formation of a planned, experimental tear (Figure 3-16B) as the axis of the loops is dialed into the region of the tear (Figures 3-16C to 16E). As long as the loops are perpendicular to the tear (situated in distant quadrants such as shown in Figures 3-16B and C), the danger is less. This is clearly the mechanism that is responsible for some clinical decentrations. Recalling again that decentration is one of the major nagging complications of this surgical procedure, attention to performing an anterior capsulectomy without creation of radial tears assumes greater importance.

Conclusion

Figure 3-17 illustrates how a well-implanted, in-the-bag posterior chamber IOL can be snugly, securely, and permanently set in place behind an intact anterior capsule. Modern IOLs, built more and more to conform to the size and shape of the capsular bag (Figure 3-18), implanted with

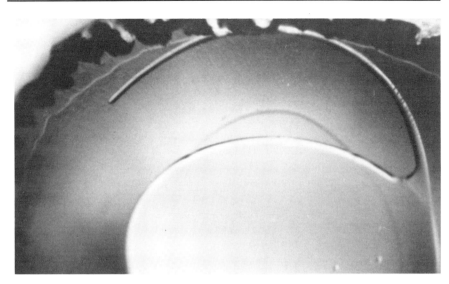

Figure 3-17: Oblique view into the anterior segment of a human eye obtained post-mortem in which an experimental capsulorhexis, hydrodissection, phacoemulsification and insertion of a 12.0 mm. one piece modified C-loop PC-IOL has been implanted. This view through a scleral window shows a well centered IOL and the loops are securely fastened between the anterior capsular remnant and posterior capsule. No problems would be expected in such a case.

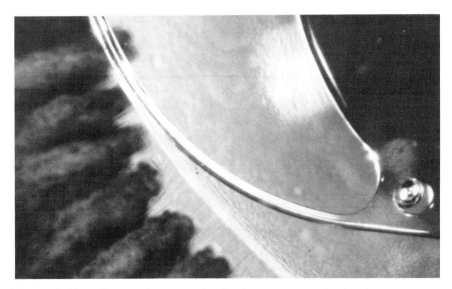

Figure 3-18: Gross photograph of a human eye obtained post-mortem in which a well manufactured 13.5 mm. one piece all PMMA modified C-loop PC-IOL has been implanted following capsulorhexis, hydrodissection and phacoemulsification. Note the excellent conformation of the loops sandwiched between the posterior capsule and intact, sufficiently large anterior capsular flap.

modern anterior capsulectomy techniques such as CCC and hydrodissection, should further decrease the incidence of significant clinical complications such as decentration.

References

1. Neuhann T: Theorie and Operationstecknik der Kapsulorhexis. Klin Monatsbl Augenheilkd, 190:542–545, 1987.
2. Gimbel, HV, Neuhann T: Development, advantages and methods of the continuous circular capsulorhexis technique. J. Cat. Refract Surg. 16 (1): 31–37, 1990.
3. Apple DJ, Kincaid MC, Mamalis N, Olson RJ: *Intraocular Lenses. Evolution, Designs, Complications, and Pathology.* Baltimore, Williams & Wilkins, 1989.
4. Apple DJ, Tetz MR, Hansen SO, McKnight GT, Richards SC, Brems RN, and Yeomans MM: Intercapsular implantation of various posterior chamber IOLs: animal test results, Ophthalmic Practice 5(3):100–104 and 132–134, 1987.
5. Davison, JA: Analysis of capsular bag defect and intraocular lens positions for consistent centration. J. Cat. Refract. Surg. 12:124–129, 1986.
6. Wasserman D, Apple DJ, Castaneda VE, and associates: Anterior capsular tears and loop fixation of posterior chamber intraocular lenses (submitted to Ophthalmology).
7. Apple DJ, Park SB, Merkely KH, Brems RN, Richards SC, Langley KE, Piest KL, and Isenberg RA: Posterior chamber intraocular lenses in a series of 75 autopsy eyes. Part I: Loop location, J. Cat. Refract. Surg. 12:358–362, 1986.
8. McDonnell PJ, Champion R, and Green WR: Location and composition of haptics of posterior chamber intraocular lenses: histological study of postmortem eyes, Ophthalmology 94:136–142, 1987.
9. Apple DJ, Lim ES, Morgan RC, Tsai JC, Gwin TD, Brown SJ, Carlson AN: Preparation and study of human eyes obtained postmortem with the Miyake posterior photographic technique, Ophthalmology 97:810–816, 1990.
10. Hansen SO, Tetz MR, Solomon KD, Borup MD, Brems RN, O'Morchoe DJC, Bouhaddou O, Apple DJ: Decentration of flexible loop posterior chamber intraocular lenses in a series of 222 postmortem eyes, Ophthalmology 95(3):344–349, 1988.
11. Brems RN, Apple DJ, Pfeffer BR, Park SB, Piest KL, and Isenberg RA: Posterior chamber intraocular lenses in a series of 75 autopsy eyes. Part III: Correlation of positioning holes and optic edges with the pupillary aperture and visual axis, J. Cat. Refract. Surg. 12:367–371, 1986.
12. Assia EI, Apple DJ, Tsai JC, and associates: Mechanism of Radial tear formation and extension after anterior capsulectomy, (submitted to Ophthalmology).

13. Assia EI, Apple DJ, Gwin TD, and associates: A comparative experimental surgical study of various anterior capsulectomy techniques, (submitted to Arch. Ophthalmol).
14. Rosen E. (ed.): Special issue on capsular surgery. Eur. J. Implant. Ref. Surg, March(2):1–88, 1990.

Chapter 4

ROUNDTABLE DISCUSSION CURRENT TECHNIQUES OF CAPSULORHEXIS

Howard V. Gimbel, MD, Moderator

Gimbel: I would like to start this roundtable discussion on capsulorhexis by talking about the size of opening I perform. I like to have the capsular edge—the opening—smaller than the diameter of the implant. The reason for this is I have seen that when the anterior capsule adheres to the posterior capsule, it seems to be the stimulus for fibrosis to develop and spread across the posterior capsule or contract the posterior capsule into folds. Also, I have seen particularly in sulcus placed implants, but occasionally in a shallow chamber case, that the iris will stick to the posterior capsule much more easily than to the anterior capsule. So, I like to have the posterior capsule all covered with anterior capsule. I have seen a contracture of the edge and for that reason, also, I like to have that contracture occur in front of the whole diameter of the implant rather than on one side only, and then catch the edge of the implant on another side which may nudge it to one side. A smaller capsulorhexis allows purse string contracture over the anterior surface of the lens which is a complication you may see, and I'm wondering if any of the faculty have seen similar complications from capsulorhexis.

Hunkeler: I've seen the collapse of the ring and contracture of the ring, especially in younger patients and patients who are predisposed with preexisting, mild inflammatory disease—arthritic patients—and it can be a perplexing problem. It is a problem, but the treatment is to do a YAG anterior capsulotomy. For those of you have not done it, it is a relatively easy procedure to perform with essentially no damage to the implant. It is not a significant problem. You can do a series of relaxing incisions to allow the ring to relax back. My personal feeling is that the capsulectomy needs to be right at 5 mm, and in my mind's eye I can picture a drawing by Duke Elder showing where the anterior capsule is the very thickest—and that is just central to the insertion of the zonules on the anterior surface of the anterior capsule. That is where the capsule is the thickest, so if you can stay within that zone I think you are going to have the most solid circular or continuous ring. That's why I prefer to have it there. The other thing is that I would like to put it there to start with rather than starting out with a smaller capsulectomy, because I don't know that I'm going to have the ability to go back—because of a number of reasons—after the lens implant insertion, and enlarge the capsulectomy. I'd prefer, if at all possible, to make it just exactly the shape that I want when I make the initial pass. Among other things, it also saves some time doing it that way.

Roberts: One of the things that I'm concerned about is the insertion point of the zonules into the anterior capsule. As you know, the zonules don't insert at the equator, but they insert anteriorly, and when you make the capsulorhexis a little bit too big it is quite easy to disinsert some zonules and it kind of defeats the purpose of the capsulorhexis which is to prevent decentration. I think that my capsulorhexis is a little bit larger than Dr. Gimbel's. I'm probably just not as good at making it as he is, and therefore it tends to enlarge. I've never had the problem, consequently, of having the ring contract because it is big. One of the things that I do notice is that in the situations where the capsulorhexis is larger than the implant, I get fibrosis of the anterior capsule to the posterior capsule and maybe that is a small barrier to decentration.

Gimbel: I think that's true. As I mentioned, though, if you get that on one side but the capsular rim is covering the implant on the other side, that's when I think that the implant could be nudged to one side. If it is outside the diameter of the implant all the way around, that could well be true. Hal?

Balyeat: I would just like to make a suggestion for those people who primarily do planned extracapsular surgery. I wouldn't rush out and start doing a lot of capsulorhexis procedures if you are doing planned extracapsular surgery. My experience has been that if you have the right size capsulorhexis, it works fine. If your capsulorhexis is just a little bit small or the nucleus is a little bit large, then the force of the vectors at play will cause the capsulorhexis or the anterior capsule to tear—usually in one spot, and it's usually at 12 o'clock—one of the places you would rather not have it tear before you start your cortical cleanup. So, in my experience in most cases it is preferable to do a can opener technique with a planned extracapsular procedure. The other admonition, perhaps, is the size of the capsulorhexis when you are using a 6.5–7 mm lens. It is very difficult to get those lenses, particularly the one piece lenses, into the bag if your capsulorhexis is too small. After you have done a very nice small capsulorhexis and you've done a phacoemulsification in the bag, for instance, and then you have a capsulorhexis that is too small, then you end up with your lens in the ciliary sulcus and you really have defeated the purpose. So, I'm interested in the technique of enlarging the capsular opening.

Gimbel: I would like to present the other side of the argument in regard to extracapsular surgery, because I've had people question me on this.

It's my view that with extracapsular surgery, capsulorhexis should be done and when necessary purposeful relaxing incisions in the rim may be made before nucleus removal. Although I do very little extracapsular surgery now, but when I do have a dense, brunescent, rock hard nucleus that I feel is too risky to phacoemulsify, I will still do a capsulorhexis but do the relaxing incisions purposefully at 10 and 2 o'clock superiorly, loop out the lens, and then after lens implantation put the implant in and again make inferiorly matching incisions. You mentioned a tear at 12 o'clock where you don't want it, but I'd rather have one at 12 o'clock or 10 and 2 o'clock than one at 6 o'clock as I put the lens implant in.

Balyeat: I would agree that if you do the relaxing incisions, that that will take care of that problem. I think the benefit to having a rim, even if it's only the lower half, is that the lower part of the capsule is very resistant to the force that has to be applied when you put the loops into the bag.

Gimbel: John?

Hunkeler: By putting those two relaxing incisions in, you are doing essentially an envelope or intracapsular procedure, bypassing and avoiding the need to go back and remove the anterior capsule in the procedure, which again, if you have any positive posterior pressure or for whatever reason a shallowing of the chamber, that makes it very difficult to go back and grasp that capsule flap and do that procedure. I would like to avoid that. I don't see the value of going back to do something that you could have done earlier in the operation. I think it is a waste of time and it adds an increased risk for the patient—going back in to do something that if you had designed the operation properly, you would have done it from the start.

Gimbel: I agree. I also like to make it the size and the position that I want initially, but in certain circumstances such as poor visualization, I use this technique. It's a pretty rare event, intumescent cases, but in most cases I do like to purposefully make it small.

Hunkeler: Probably the best thing to tell everybody is that watching the video of Howard doing these capsulorhexis procedures (without viscoelastic substance), is showing state of the art, as in the saying "It don't get any better than that." Howard does this extremely well and has experience now up to six years. I tried to do it that way without using viscoelastic and was not very successful. After listening to Howard and Tom Neuhann and a few other people, I finally realized that the only way I was going to be able to do it effectively—and the reason I'm saying this is that to try and do it without a viscoelastic is very difficult. I found that I had to use a viscoelastic, keep the chamber deep, and adequately flatten the convexity of the anterior surface of the lens. Usually, if you say something correct then you get the nods.

Cal and Howard are nodding, but if you let the anterior surface of the lens come up—either because of positive posterior pressure, elasticity in a younger patient, or whatever—you will almost be guaranteed to get a radial tear in spite of all your diligent efforts to bring the tear in the center. It will go posteriorly. So, if that starts happening you have to add more viscoelastic. That's why I got into using the visoelastic to start with, and then developed a technique that basically tries to do exactly the same thing that Howard is doing, but doing it with a viscoelastic. For those of you who are interested in beginning the procedure, I strongly encourage you to use a viscoelastic. Cal may be able to comment. We'll see if he agrees. I want to congratulate Howard on developing the technique and Tom Neuhann as well, for doing it as well as they do. It gives a role for all of us to emulate.

Roberts: I certainly use a viscoelastic and I think I cheat a little bit from the purists, because I start out with Vannas scissors to start my capsulotomy, and I make a cut which is maybe two or three clock hours which gets me going in the right direction. Then, I come in with my capsulorhexis forceps and complete it. For me, I find that the hardest part of the procedure is the first couple of clock hours getting started. I find that the easiest part is down below and goes from 7 o'clock to 5 o'clock as I do it left handed. So, by using the scissors, it gets me started before I continue it with the forceps, making the rest much easier. When I tried to do it with a small puncture and then grab the capsule, the capsulorhexis immediately went out to the equator. Moreover, it was hard for me to get started and that's when I began having posterior capsule tears that I wasn't looking forward to having.

Gimbel: One thing that I would ask you about though, is when you make that scissors snip and you get radial tears, are they quite likely to be where you've made that scissors snip at 12 o'clock? I think it probably is very difficult to get a very smooth edge with a scissors snip, the same as Tom Neuhann with his needle puncture which is a slit that he tears both ways. He admits that sometimes it isn't a perfect slit and will tear there. He is going more to starting centrally as well, like the rest of us.

Roberts: My cut is not superiorly. My cut is laterally. So, it is a vertical type of cut that goes on the side . . .

Gimbel: But it is in the radius of your tear though?

Roberts: Correct.

Gimbel: It is very smooth edged and doesn't have any tendency to tear at that point?

Roberts: It really doesn't. With a nice long angled Vannas scissors you get a nice clean tear.

Gimbel: That's interesting. I want to respond, before I forget, to John's comments about viscoelastic. I agree. I think that to develop the technique and learn the vector forces and so forth, certainly viscoelastic is advantageous. But, if you had used a viscoelastic in that intumescent case—which is the case you think you need it in because of the positive pressure and so forth—what happens is that milky fluid just clouds the viscoelastic and you can't see anything. I've had that experience, and that's why I've gone back to just an irrigating cystotome with balanced salt irrigation for those liquid cortex cases. You can just sit there for a few minutes and let the irrigation wash out the milky fluid that is exuding, and then once it quits clouding your view, proceed. If it keeps coming again, you stop and let it irrigate. On occasion, with a very soft lens, I've just made a little slit like that centrally, and this milky fluid keeps coming and coming so I've taken the cystotome out and started aspirating with a 27–30 gauge cannula, and aspirated to get rid of the whole lens just with aspiration through a cannula. I then proceeded with the capsulorhexis after the lens was removed through a little slit-like opening. So, viscoelastics are good but there are some circumstances where they will impede your view. I have found also, as you noted there, when the viscoelastics are in the eye it is kind of hard to grasp the capsule. The viscosity keeps moving it away from you. If you have a very, very soft eye—I think that is key to this too, to have a good retrobulbar, no extraocular muscle movement and a pressure device on long enough to have a soft eye—that will make your capsulorhexis much, much easier. The difficulty in the technique is when you have positive vitreous pressure. This pressure must be neutralized with viscoelastics. So, just a few points on that. Did you want to respond, John?

Hunkeler: I was just going to say, that there is a gentle change in the surgical technique with phacoemulsification. Many of the early phacoemulsifier proponents did not use ocular pressure and wanted the positive pressure to bring the nucleus upward. Although we didn't go into it, with the emulsification technique that you eloquently showed, you really don't want that positive pressure to bring the nucleus forward. Whereas, previously, a lot of surgeons did prefer to have the nucleus come forward. Certainly, if you prefer to have the nucleus come forward—much as I do—I don't spend as much time with ocular pressure. I want a little positive pressure to do the phacoemulsification at the aperture opening in the capsulorhexis plane. So, I have to use a viscoelastic. It was obvious from the videos and from listening to what you said, that the eye was much softer than what I am accustomed to having and it's just a difference in technique.

Gimbel: That's right. Little things like that you don't think about sometimes ahead of time, but it becomes obvious.

Hunkeler: Yes. Let me just say one other thing. I was interested to hear the new term "continuous circular capsulorhexis." Let me just put a little pitch in to maybe somehow get rid of the term "continuous" because I think a lot of people when they get into doing the procedure think of the word "continuous" and think you have to do it all in one fell swoop. You really don't. It's actually regrasping and making continual changes rather than doing it all in one continuous pass. If you try to do that, the success rate I guarantee would not be quite as great as it is by regrasping or repositioning the instrument to get a better position during the process.

Gimbel: I hadn't thought about that. I thought of the term "continuous" because the tear has no end. It's one tear that continues all the way around. Mathematicians use the term "continuous curve" for closed loops such as ovals, ellipses, and circles. That's the reason for the term as it is.

Hunkeler: The reason I say that is you get in your mind that you are supposed to do it all in one pass.

Gimbel: That's a good point.

Hunkeler: If you think of a word and don't translate it correctly to your hands, you may end up getting in trouble.

Gimbel: Well, I think it is important though to add at least "circular" or something, because capsulorhexis only means to tear the capsule, and we all know that certain tears of the capsule we try not to get.

Hunkeler: Mine are never perfect circles like yours.

Gimbel: Mine aren't always either. I just show the perfect circles!

Roberts: The best tip that was given to me on doing capsulorhexis, was to think about always folding the capsule over on top of itself and continuing it that way. Using the technique that you showed, was when I started getting better circles.

Gimbel: Yes. That's a contribution Tom Neuhann has made to this technique. As I showed you however, I don't find it advantageous in every section of the tear. It's interesting that for me it works better, as I said, when I'm pushing or going away from the wound with the tear. And yet, when I'm coming toward the wound with the tear, then I like to get on the anterior surface or hooking the side of it or something. Hal?

Balyeat: Yes, back to planned extracapsular surgery. I find it interesting the way ophthalmology evolves and the way that techniques that are good seem to finally be incorporated into cataract surgery. I suspect that capsulorhexis will be one of those. I think in a perfect world, at least in my experience, if I do a phacoemulsification with a capsulorhexis and have an implant in the bag, that is a very nice if not a perfect operation for me. But, the 7 mm lens gives us a fair amount of leeway in terms of our capsule—something that we didn't have before when we were using smaller lenses. Certainly, if small incision surgery and foldable lenses or small, ovoid lenses become the norm in the future, then the capsulorhexis is going to be terribly critical to the performance of a good procedure, because we are going to be back to the way we used to be where we didn't quite know where the lenses were. We were using 6 or 6.5mm lenses with all kinds of holes and whistles and bells on the haptics, and the decentration problem was very serious. Most of us had patients complaining of glare in many cases, particularly in dim light. With a 7mm lens, certainly if you do a can opener technique or if you have problems with the capsule, you are much less likely to have a problem. I don't think that people should leave this morning with the impression that capsulorhexis is the only thing that you should do and that everybody ought to be doing capsulorhexis. I think that there is a lot to be said for a good planned extracapsular operation with a can opener technique and a 7 mm lens. I don't think that people should feel badly in any way, if that is the technique that they use and use very well.

Gimbel: That brings up another thought on the size of the capsulorhexis. As many of you have probably witnessed, when the anterior capsule fuses to the posterior capsule you get some slight translucency instead of transparency. I think that is an advantage also, keeping the anterior capsule opening smaller than the implant, so that if it covers the edge of the implant and I think would reduce any glare if there might be glare from its edge. This principle might allow us to use the 5.5 mm with little concern about the edge glare, because of the way the peripheral capsule opacifies a bit and actually covers the edge of the implant. That is just theoretical, but Charlie Kelman said to me after my presentation on the two-stage capsulorhexis at the ASCRS last year, "Well, you should just leave it that small and put in a 5mm diameter lens and let it opacify and it will be just like my Phaco-fit lens. You don't have to enlarge it and put in a big lens; just use a little lens and let the capsule cover the edge." John?

Hunkeler: I would agree with what Charlie said and also with what Hal said about planned extracapsular surgery. Certainly for those patients where a planned extracapsular surgery is the only choice, that's what I do, but the vast majority of patients end up receiving phacoemulsification. With the increasing experience with the capsulorhexis technique, there is no question in my mind that you get a higher level of accurate centration of the intraocular lens. I question the need to have a 7 mm intraocular lens and even question in many cases the need for a 6mm diameter intraocular lens. With the foldable technology that is proving quite successful, we are able to take advantage of phacoemulsification and, much as Dr. Gimbel has said, one of the key steps in that is the capsulorhexis. It is a little out of sequence to be talking about it right now. I think probably the first thing to talk about is making the proper incision, but we now have the potential in cataract surgery to get prompt visual rehabilitation and I think that is going to become an increasing issue for patients and for the physicians as well.

Gimbel: Something I would like to say to those of you doing extracapsular surgery, is that a lot of techniques are coming along to allow for extracapsular surgery with capsulorhexis, even in the smaller openings that we have been talking about. Those are the hydrodissection and hydrodelamination—separating out the densest part of the nucleus, away from the epinucleus—and Dr. Luther Fry's technique of sort of stripping the epinucleus off the nucleus as he pulls it through a small incision. This technique cannot be used for the softer nuclei, and we now seem to be doing cataract surgery at an earlier stage. I think this allows for extracapsular surgery to be done with the same capsulorhexis opening and even smaller scleral incisions, while still maintaining that circular opening in the capsule. Certainly, in the very dense brunescent cases, we have to make a larger capsulectomy other than capsulorhexis, or else make controlled relaxing cuts in the capsulorhexis rim. Thank you very much to our panelists.

Chapter 5

EVOLVING IN THE CAPSULE TECHNIQUE OF PHACOEMULSIFICATION

Howard V. Gimbel, MD

In 1974 participants of the Fourth Annual David J. Kelman Research Foundation Meeting voted to recognize Charles Kelman as the Father of Phacoemulsification. His procedure was officially named Kelman Phacoemulsification (KPE).[2] Phacoemulsification had found its place in ophthalmology because of its immeasurable benefit to the patient. Since its development in 1967 by Kelman, phacoemulsification techniques have been evolving in order to meet the challenges of extracapsular cataract extraction. In-situ nucleofractis is the latest advance in the more ideal small incision surgery with posterior chamber (PC) in-the-bag intraocular lens (IOL) implantation.

The origins of Kelman's phacoemulsification has been described in the literature in detail.[2] Kelman's original technique involved the use of a 15 degree angle ultrasound tip. His preference was to perform phacoemulsification in the anterior chamber. As technology evolved, so did the technique. Kelman began giving courses on KPE. Robert M. Sinskey in the early 1970's developed a technique of using KPE in the posterior chamber. By 1973 he developed basically an "in the bag" one-handed technique. Instead of delivering the nucleus into the anterior chamber, he used a 15 degree phaco tip for sculpting the central nucleus down posteriorly almost to the posterior capsule before removing the peripheral nuclear shell. Sinskey still uses this technique but with a 45 degree phaco tip.

Jared Emery and James Little also showed early interest in KPE.[2] Little's interest was more clinical and he developed his own variation of nuclear sculpting. His technique involved partial in-the-bag and partial in the anterior chamber emulsification. Little proceeded with sculpting of the central anterior nucleus using a 45 degree phaco tip. He then tilted the remaining nucleus and prolapsed it out at the superior equator into the anterior chamber. Emulsification was thus largely carried out in the pupillary space between the cornea and the posterior chamber. Little also introduced the use of a second instrument while doing KPE. To help maneuver the nucleus, he passed a spatula into the anterior chamber along side the phaco tip through the 12 o'clock incision (Knolle, G. Ophthalmology Times, Nov. 15/89, p. 23).

Richard P. Kratz popularized two-handed KPE by using a spatula through a second side port incision at 3 o'clock. Guy E. Knolle, Jr. built on Little's technique of partial in-the-bag/partial anterior chamber emulsification. Using a 45 degree phaco tip, he sculpted the central nucleus with subsequent prolapse of the 9 o'clock equator. Knolle then used counterclockwise rotation for mostly in the posterior capsule emulsification.

I first began using phacoemulsification in 1974. In 1975 I combined KPE with Binkhorst 2 loop iridocapsular lens implants. I became more confident and comfortable with KPE than with planned extracapsular or intercapsular cataract extraction (ECCE/ICCE) for all except the extremely brunescent cataracts and lenses with little or no zonular support. My KPE techniques have varied from those originally taught by Dr. Kelman at his course in 1974. Some changes I had learned from Dr. Richard Kratz, and Dr. Robert Sinskey, and others from Dr. James Little, and still others have evolved from my own experience and innovation. My accumulated experience through February 1990 was 24,877 cases (Gimbel Eye Centre Statistics).

In the late 1970's, I began to make the transition from Kelman's original prolapsing of the nucleus out of the capsule into the anterior chamber to techniques which tipped up the upper pole of the lens for emulsification in the posterior chamber. Very soft nuclei were difficult to prolapse into the chamber and tip up for emulsification. These cataracts of younger patients stimulated the transition into in-situ or in-the-bag phacoemulsification. As I used this technique for more dense cataracts, and being accustomed to using a second instrument as taught by Kratz, I developed fracturing techniques to allow for phacoemulsification within the capsular bag in more mature cataracts.

In the early 1980's, as the technique evolved to application for mature and very dense nuclei, it became evident that the nuclear fracturing techniques not only made it possible to do phacoemulsification within the capsular bag, but added to the safety of the procedure for dense nuclei and made KPE of these cataracts much more efficient.

I first began using "Divide and Conquer" in-situ phacoemulsification in 1986. The technique had evolved because of one basic concept: it was easier to emulsify a cataract that was systematically divided and fragmented rather than impale the nucleus in a randomized fashion.

In-situ or endolenticular Divide and Conquer Nucleofractis phacoemulsification is so named because of its efficiency and efficacy in challenging cases such as dense brunescent nuclei and small pupils. The nucleus is "conquered" by fragmenting or fracturing it into pieces, for which I have coined the term "nucleo-fractis". The technique was developed to give an increased efficiency to phacoemulsification and to extend phaco to very hard nuclei. The Divide and Conquer technique was introduced first in September 1987 in Jerusalem for the European Intraocular Implant Lens Council, and then via a video presentation at the 1988 Canadian Rockies Symposium on Cataract and Refractive Surgery in Calgary, Alberta.

Modifications of nucleofractis can be used for almost the entire spectrum of lens opacities including intumescent and brunescent lenses, but exempting the very soft nucleus of young people and the posterior subcapsular opacities with quite soft nuclei of the middle-aged. Nucleofractis has allowed me to use phacoemulsification in almost 100% of my cases. In a series of 7,174 consecutive cataract cases, 99.8% were accomplished by phaco.[3] In only 0.1% did I have to use ECCE or ICCE because of very weak zonules or cataracta nigra.

I begin my surgical method by making a limbus based conjunctival flap which I suture securely closed at the end of the procedure. Episcleral vessels are cauterized using bipolar tip cautery that has little tendency to shrink or char tissue. A routine paracentesis is made with a 45 degree diamond knife which allows for

1. Two-handed phaco technique
2. Iris/capsular bag manipulation with bent cannula or spatula
3. Right angle bimanual control/assistance for IOL insertion/placement
4. Insertion and removal of viscoelastics, air, BSS.

The paracentesis should be made approximately at 70–90 degrees from the centre of the phaco incision to provide optimum position for pivoting the cyclodialysis spatula or irrigation cannula for maneuvers within the eye. These maneuvers can be done through either the paracentesis incision or the corneal-scleral incision to reach any position of the anterior chamber and lens capsule.

I use the posterior limbal Acute Bevelled Cataract (ABC) corneal-scleral incision. There is good astigmatism management with this incision.[4]

Using Continuous Circular Capsulorhexis (CCC) or Two-Staged CCC to make a small capsulectomy, I then proceed with two-handed in-situ Divide and Conquer nuclear cracking or nucleofractis phacoemulsification except in soft lenses. CCC is a prerequisite to doing Divide and Conquer nucleofractis, because in many ways one technique demands the other.[7] The nucleus is left in the lens capsule at all times with phaco done entirely within the capsular bag. The classical divide and conquer should only be attempted where there are no anterior capsule tears because cracking the nuclear rim in the capsule will almost certainly cause extensions of these tears. CCC produces a resilient smooth-edged capsulectomy that prevents tags or flaps, and resists anterior capsule tears during this maneuver. If an anterior capsule tear is present, I still use two-handed in-the-bag phaco but carefully emulsify the first section of the nuclear rim. Then there is space for subsequent cracking without stretching the capsular rim.

Once CCC is achieved, I proceed with hydrodissection just under the anterior capsule using a 3cc syringe and a 30g cannula. I attempt to separate the cortex or at least the epi-nucleus from the capsule and peripheral cortex. In dense cataracts, and particularly if the zonules are weak, I do thorough hydrodissection until the lens can be rotated within the capsular bag using the 30 g cannula. To avoid rupturing the capsule from the fluid pressure, I wash out anterior cortical material just under the capsule over a wide arc before attempting to force fluid behind the nucleus so that there is no restriction to this fluid getting out of the capsule as it dissects posteriorly, then anteriorly again. The wound must be distended enough with the cannula to allow fluid to escape from the anterior chamber. I avoid using this technique in cases of posterior lenticonus because of the risks of central posterior capsule rupture. I perform complete hydrodissection with entry through the paracentesis to reach the 12 o'clock area until the lens can be rotated within the capsular bag. Completeness of hydrodissection is verified by easy rotation of the nucleus within the capsule. As part of the bimanual technique, the freed nucleus is then stabilized using a cyclodialysis spatula through the paracentesis and emulsification can begin.

There are four basic steps to Divide and Conquer In-Situ Nucleofractis Phacoemulsification:

1. Deep central coring of lens material until a donut of thick nuclear rim and, if any, only a very thin posterior plate of nuclear material remains
2. Cracking or fracturing the nuclear rim to break away a pie-shaped section
3. Rotation of the nuclear rim for further nucleofractis until the nuclear rim is divided into 4 to 8 sections
4. Emulsification of each pie-shaped sections or nuclear sub-units

The central part of the nucleus is emulsified by a sculpting technique continuing posteriorly until the central nucleus is actually entirely removed down to the epi-nuclear material posteriorly. This leaves a nuclear rim which then can be fractured using a bimanual technique. After the first crack, the lens is rotated and a section is broken away by creating another adjacent crack or fracture. Nucleofractis is continued until the lens is fully rotated and fractured into pie-shaped sections. These sections can then be brought into the central area of the capsule and pupil for efficient and safe emulsification. At present, I have developed six nucleofractis styles, variations of which can be used depending on the density of the lens nucleus.

STYLE #1 Very Hard Mature Brunescent Cataracts
  —use small CCC or Two Staged CCC
  —insist on all nuclear cracking first in order to stabilize last nuclear section for cracking

A mature lens best demonstrates Divide and Conquer Nucleofractis graphically. There should be no tug on the zonules during rotation of the nucleus after hydrodissection. The phaco tip is used to carve or core out a deep crater in the centre of the nucleus (Figure 5-1). Emulsification is initiated at a point slightly right of centre and coring is accomplished between 11–7 o'clock. As the tip approaches the posterior capsule revealing the pink retinal reflex, less and less ultrasound power is used. The danger of perforating the posterior capsule is significantly reduced if a shaving action of the phaco tip, never an impaling one, is used while coring the deep nuclear layers. Complete coring will show the pink reflex centrally.

It is necessary to make the crater wide enough to easily accommodate not only the phaco tip but also the silicone irrigation sleeve. The nucleus is displaced inferiorly to thin the superior part and then to the left to extend the coring to the right.

When nuclear material is no longer accessible from the initial position, the nucleus is rotated clockwise and additional nuclear shaving performed. This procedure is repeated until as much of the central core of the lens as possible has been removed, leaving an intact rim of nucleus which keeps the capsule uniformly stretched.

For mature lenses, I like to leave the nuclear sections in place before emulsifying any of them, but they can be emulsified one by one as soon as they are isolated. Leaving them in place maintains the architecture of the capsular bag and facilitates nucleofractis.

Systematic nucleofractis is begun by cracking the remaining nuclear donut at the 5 to 6 o'clock position. This is accomplished by the bimanual technique. With a short burst of ultrasound the 15 degree or 30 degree phaco tip is burrowed into the peripheral nucleus and held there with

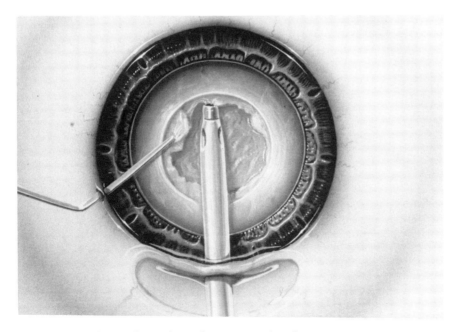

Figure 5-1:   Central carving of a mature hard cataract.

suction using foot position two. For right-handed surgeons, the cyclodialysis spatula is used to stabilize or apply pressure to the left while the phaco tip applies pressure to the right (Figure 5-2). In this way nucleofractis of the nuclear rim and posterior nucleus is achieved at the 5–6 o'clock position.

With the nuclear rim fragmented, emulsification of these subunits may begin. Nuclear sections are brought into the centre of the capsule and pupil for efficient emulsification with good control of the fragments (Figure 5-3). First a short burst of low power ultrasound is used to engage one of the sections. While maintaining suction only, this section will fold into the center of the pupil if the central posterior nucleus has been thinned sufficiently. Once in the center of the lens and positioned below or posterior to the plane of the iris, emulsification can be performed safely with turbulence contained within the capsular bag.

After the first section is removed, subsequent sections are brought to the centre and emulsified, rotating the entire nucleus clockwise or counterclockwise a few degrees each time. If a portion of the lens will not fold into the centre, further thinning of the posterior central nucleus may be required. Here the central lens material may have been weakened but not completely broken by nucleofractis and may require additional separation. The spatula may be used to lift a thin layer of posterior nucleus up to the phaco port.

To avoid contact between the posterior capsule and the phaco tip as the last few fragments are emulsified, the tip should be kept well above

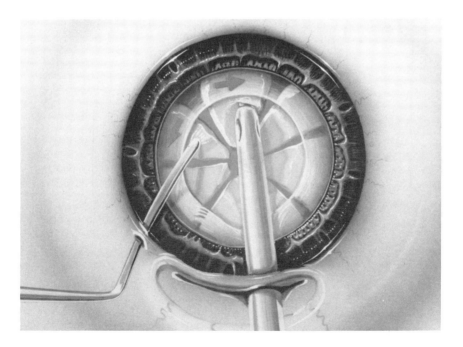

Figure 5-2:   Right-handed bimanual crater divide and conquer nucleofractis.

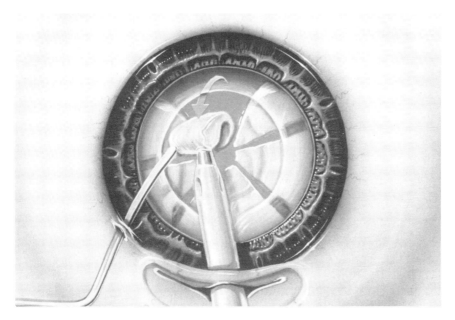

Figure 5-3:   Nuclear sections are brought into the center of the capsule for efficient emulsification.

the posterior capsule, maneuvering the lens material to the center using the cyclodialysis spatula along with suction and very short bursts of phaco. Low power ultrasound phaco is used and the posterior capsule is watched carefully because it can unexpectedly come up and make contact with the phaco tip because it no longer has nuclear rim holding it posteriorly. To further protect the posterior capsule, the spatula is placed just under the tip so that it will hold the capsule back in case there is an anterior movement of the posterior capsule when a lens fragment enters the port. Each section of lens material to be emulsified is stabilized with the spatula to keep it within the pupillary plane in order to avoid endothelial touch and phaco turbulence near the cornea.

In very dense brunescent lenses I use moderately high phaco power for the shaving technique to core out the central part of the lens. Again turbulence is contained down inside the bowl of the capsular bag and not directed at the cornea. After coring, a cross-instrument action technique is used when doing nucleofractis. The spatula is slid across the phaco tip and pushes to the right while the phaco tip pushes left for additional leverage as these very firm nuclear rim fragments are separated. The nuclear rim of a dense brunescent cataract should be fragmented by multiple primary cracks because the smaller the sections, the more efficient and controlled in the emulsification. As the phacoemulsification nears completion, the power should be turned down so that the small hard fragments are not bounced away from the phaco tip. The spatula can be used to control any remaining firm segments so that they don't tumble up against the endothelium of the cornea.

STYLE #2 Relatively Hard Nucleus
   —involves large central coring
   —first nuclear segment (6 o'clock) emulsified just after it is broken
   away because it comes to the centre of the capsule

In relatively hard cataracts, I use divide and conquer nucleofractis after large central coring. Upon routine first and second fracturing of the nuclear rim, the first pie segment wants to come to the centre of the capsule for emulsification (Figures 5-4 and 5-5). This leaves more room to separate the other nuclear segments before removing them by emulsification. However, the latter segments are almost starting to fall into the centre before all the fracturing because of the extra room and less stability. Because these lenses are quite easy to fracture this is not a problem. This collapse of the nuclear rim demonstrates the efficiency of the Divide and Conquer technique.

In intumescent cataracts where there may be positive lens pressure and liquid cortex, I make a deliberately small CCC opening and keep the phaco tip in the centre of the opening. Rapid escape of the lens material will ensue and BSS irrigation may be required to flush the clouded anterior chamber. After this opaque lens material is removed, visualization is enhanced by the pink retinal reflex. Enlargement of the capsule opening to the desired diameter is accomplished by Two-Staged CCC.[5]

STYLE #3 Moderately Hard Nuclei
   —smaller central coring extended as trough to 6 o'clock
   —quadrant nucleofractis

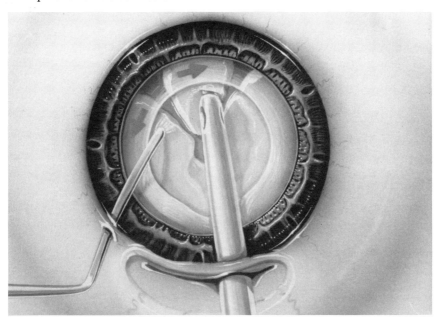

Figure 5-4: In relatively hard nuclei, the first pie segment wants to come to the center of the capsule for emulsification.

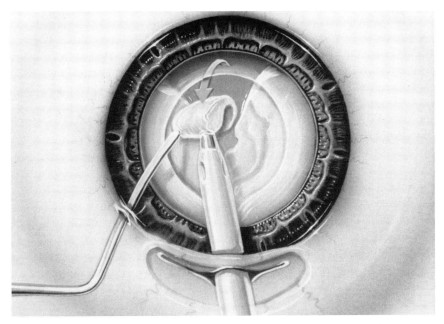

Figure 5-5:   The first pie segment is maneuvered by second instrument for emulsification, leaving a space, to help facilitate fracturing of additional segments.

In only moderately hard cataracts, I do a central but smaller coring so that enough firm nucleus remains available for fracturing. A trough is sculpted out to 6 o'clock with a routine first fracture (Figure 5-6). The second and third fractures are placed at 3 and 9 o'clock. Without rotation of the nucleus, the phaco tip engages the left hemisection at 3 o'clock and breaks away a quadrant. A second quadrant is then broken away at 9 o'clock. This leaves the upper one half of the lens to fracture after bringing it to the centre of the capsular opening. The moderately dense nuclei may be fractured into quarters or eighths. If all of the dense central nucleus is removed in the coring, there is not enough density in the rim to use the two instruments to separate and fracture.

STYLE #4 Moderately Soft Nuclei
    —no coring
    —sculpting 7 o'clock
    —hemisection emulsification

In moderately soft cataract, I break through at 7 o'clock and sculpt out the nuclear rim on the right (Figure 5-7). The left half of the cataract is left for stabilization by the spatula. Once the right half has been emulsified, the left is rotated and bisected for emulsification.

STYLE #5 Fairly Soft to Softest Nuclei
    —central trough not core
    —split soft epinucleus
    —hemisection emulsification

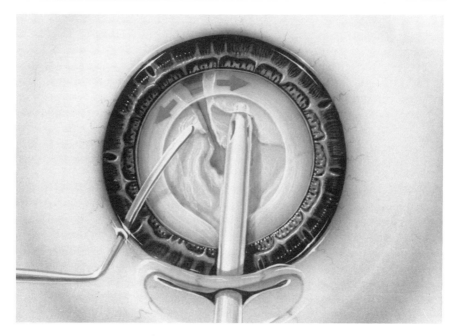

Figure 5-6: In moderately hard nuclei a trough is sculpted out to 6 o'clock with a routine first fracture.

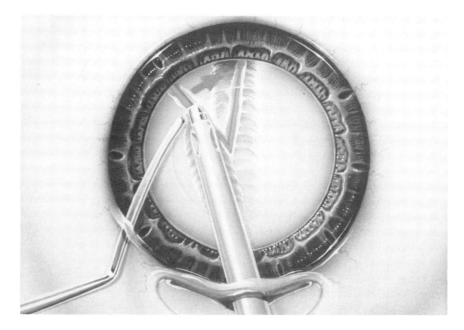

Figure 5-7: Trough Divide and Conquer Nucleofractis of moderately soft nuclei.

In soft nuclei I use a central trough to split the soft epinucleus. The trough breaks through to the periphery inferiorly while still going deep centrally. Lens material aspirates out to the periphery very easily. One has to push at the centre of the soft lens to split it before removing much of the nucleus. The first split may practically involve the entire length of the lens from top to bottom (Figure 5-8). The lens material almost falls to the centre for emulsification. Each hemisection is easily emulsified while stabilized by a second instrument. There is no special need for clock/counterclockwise rotation.

Divide and Conquer for Remaining Lens Fragments in Central Capsule

When a lens fragment is too large, nucleofractis can be used to break it into smaller sections before being emulsified (Figure 5-9). A second instrument may be used to fracture large segments into smaller ones for more efficient and controlled emulsification. This is the nucleofractis maneuvers that I first used in the early 1980's. I used these fracturing techniques long before developing the classical pie-section or pizza Divide and Conquer techniques.

John Shepherd, MD has evolved his own variation of the Divide and Conquer technique. In his two-handed procedure he creates four pie-shaped segments and brings each quadrant to the centre for emulsifi-

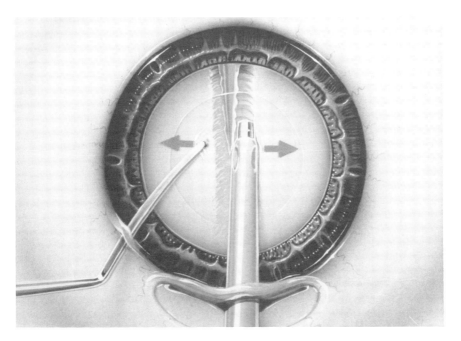

Figure 5-8:   Trough Divide and Conquer vertical split of fairly soft nuclei.

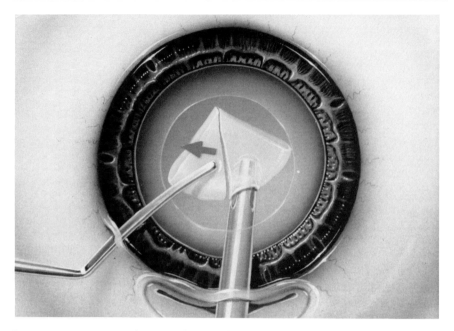

Figure 5-9: Nucleofractis of large fragment into smaller fragments.

cation. Shepherd uses hydrodissection between the capsule and nucleus and sculpts a groove from 12 to 6 o'clock. The groove is then rotated one quarter turn by the spatula and phaco tip and a cross hatched groove is then made across the original trough. The phaco tip is then placed deep in the vertical grove to stabilize the left nuclear segment while the spatula, also placed deeply, pushes away, fracturing one quadrant. The nucleus is rotated and the remaining quadrants are emulsified. The four nuclear wedges lie tightly in the capsule and are tumbled into the centre for fragmentation and easy aspiration. The phacoemulsification seems to occur in bigger chunks and is accomplished below the margin of the capsulorhexis in the posterior chamber.

Conclusion

The main principle of Divide and Conquer Nucleofractis is central coring of the nucleus with subsequent systematic nuclear rim cracking. The technique enhances the surgeon's ability for safe and efficient phacoemulsification. Modifications of the classical in-situ Divide and Conquer allow for phacoemulsification to be applied to a wide range of nuclear densities including brunescent and intumescent cataracts. Nucleofractis can be accomplished through small pupils and small capsulectomies, thereby extending KPE to glaucoma patients.[6] Together with CCC, Divide and Conquer Nucleofractis has further notable advantages. Nucleofractis is accomplished in-the-bag with reduced corneal endothelial trauma because phaco turbulence is contained within the capsular bag.[1,8] The resilient, smooth-edged rim of CCC decreases the risk of anterior capsule tears even when stretched by the phaco probe or second instrument. With an intact CCC, Nucleofractis is then safely accomplished with reduced risk of posterior capsule tears since the capsule is kept on stretch by the nuclear rim as central coring and rim fracturing is achieved. The application of Nucleofractis does have variations depending on the density of the lens, size of the pupil, intraocular hydrodynamics and the surgeon's preference. For surgeons making the transition to phacoemulsification, I recommend Nucleofractis as the technique of choice for I believe that it is easy to learn, especially when first attempted on moderately dense cataracts.

References

1. Apple DJ et al: Posterior Chamber Intraocular lens Implantation in a series of 75 autopsy eyes, Parts I-III. Journal of Cataract and Refractive Surgery, 12,1986,358–371.
2. Emery JM, Little JH: Phacoemulsification and aspiration of Cataracts, St. Louis, 1969, Mosby, ix-7.
3. Gimbel HV: Posterior Capsule Tears Using Phacoemulsification: Causes, prevention and management. Upcoming publication March 1990 European Journal of Implant and Refractive Surgery.
4. Gimbel HV: Phacoemulsification-An Instruction Manual, June 1988, p. 10.
5. Gimbel HV: Two Staged Capsulorhexis for Endocapsular Phacoemulsification. Upcoming publication Journal of Cataract and Refractive Surgery.
6. Gimbel HV, Nesbitt JAA: Small pupil: An indication for phacoemulsification. Upcoming publication Canadian Journal of Ophthalmology.
7. Gimbel HV, Neuhann T: Development, advantages and methods of the Continuous Circular Capsulorhexis technique, Journal of Cataract and Refractive Surgery, 16, 1990, 31–37.
8. Hara T, Hara T: Clinical results of endocapsular phacoemulsification and complete in-the-bag intraocular lens fixation. Journal of Cataract and Refractive Surgery, 13, 1987, 279–286.

Chapter 6

CONTROL OF CATARACT EXTRACTION

POSTOPERATIVE INTRAOCULAR PRESSURE WITH INTRACAMERAL MIOTICS

Calvin W. Roberts, MD

Intraocular pressure rises sharply in many patients immediately after cataract extraction. Though the effect is variable, the pressure may rise to 40mm.Hg. or higher.[1-18] Since the peak of pressure increase is usually in the period from six to nine hours after surgery and usually dissipates by 24 hours, routine measurement of IOP on the first post operative day will often miss the pressure spike.

Transitory increases in IOP after cataract extraction may cause pain and corneal edema, and may be a contributing factor to the development of optic nerve ischemia.[19]

Several factors may exacerbate this IOP spike. Patients with pre-existing glaucoma, even if it is well controlled, will have a higher IOP spike than non-glaucomatous patients.[20,21] The use of alpha-chymotrypsin[8,9] or sodium hyaluronate[3,11,22,23] accentuates the pressure rise. Others have suggested that tight wound closure contributes to the IOP spike.[10,24]

In an attempt to control post operative IOP spikes, many protocols have been suggested. Most surgeons irrigate sodium hyaluronate out of the anterior chamber at the end of the operation. Several pharmacologic agents used in glaucoma have proved effective in control of these pressure spikes. Acetazolamide[14] and timolol[15,25,26] have decreased the pressure rise 24 hours after intracapsular extraction. Haimann and Phelps also demonstrated the effectiveness of timolol six hours after intracapsular surgery.[4] However, after extracapsular extraction, timolol showed minimal effect on the postoperative pressure rise 24 hours after surgery.[15,27] West et al. compared the efficacy of B-blockers on early postoperative rise after extracapsular surgery and found that while levobunolol proved effective in preventing an increase in IOP, timolol and betaxolol were not statistically different from placebo.[26]

The agents most carefully studied for their effect in blunting the postoperative pressure spikes are the miotics. Both acetylcholine and carbachol, the two intraocular miotics commercially available, have been shown to be effective, though the reports are often contradictory, and the extent and duration of action differs for these two agents.[1,2,27-30] Others have studied miotics for their effect on postoperative pain, inflammation, and systemic effects.[31]

My mission today is to try to make sense out of these myriad of reports, present to you my own results from a prospective study, and present to you recommendations that you might use as a reference for the care of your patients.

Patients and Methods

40 patients scheduled for cataract extraction and posterior chamber implantation with the use of sodium hyaluronate were randomly assigned to one of two treatment groups. Group 1 received a total of 0.5 cc of acetyl choline 1.0% twice during surgery, immediately following intraocular lens placement, and at the close of the operation. The second group received placebo (BSS), also 0.5 cc according to the same protocol.

Only patients with normal intraocular pressures and no clinically significant disease in either eye, apart from cataracts, were eligible. Patients were excluded if they had previous ocular surgery, uveitis, a chronic need for ocular medication or if they had insulin dependent diabetes. As our cataract surgery is routinely performed on an ambulatory basis, the patients had to be willing to stay overnight to be studied.

All surgery was performed by the same surgeon using the same preoperative, operative, and postoperative procedures in all patients. All patients received 75 mg of indomethacin by mouth the morning of their operation. Pupil dilation was achieved with three sets of 2.5% phenylephrine and 2% cyclopentalate 15 minutes apart. Intravenous sedation was achieved with midazolam (1–3 mg) and alfentanil (250–500 mg). A modified Van Lindt (5cc) and retrobulbar block (2cc) was given with a combination mixture of 2% lidocaine with epinephrine and 0.75% bupivicaine. A Honan balloon at a pressure of 30 mmHg. was applied to the eye for twenty minutes. A standard manual extracapsular cataract extraction was performed and a 6 mm. no holes Sinskey type intraocular lens with 10% angled prolene haptics was implanted in all patients. Sodium hyaluronate was used in all patients prior to making the capsulectomy and prior to implantation of the intraocular lens. It was then aggressively irrigated out of the anterior chamber prior to the injection of the miotic or control solution. No intracameral epinephrine was used on any patient. The surgical wound was closed watertight with 6 interrupted sutures of 10-0 nylon sutures. Gentamicin drops were instilled beneath the sterile patch. No subconjunctival injections were given.

The patients were examined preoperatively, at the end of the operation, and then at three, six, nine, and 24 hours after surgery. At each examination intraocular pressure was measured in the supine position with the same Goldmann type applanation tonometer, the corneal thickness was measured with the same ultrasonic pachymeter, and the pupil was measured horizontally and vertically. The examiner making the measurements was not the operating surgeon and was blinded as to which group the patient was in.

There was no difference between the 20 subjects enrolled in the acetyl choline group and the 20 patients enrolled in the control group with respect to age, sex, race, and iris color.

Mean and mean change from baseline for IOP, pupil size (horizontal and vertical) and pachymetry were compared between groups at the end of surgery, and at 3, 6, 9, and 24 hours post surgery using a group t test. Within treatment group, changes from baseline were evaluated using a paired t test.

Results

Table 6-1 lists the mean and standard deviation of intraocular pressure, pupil diameter and corneal thickness at each point of examination. The same data is displayed graphically in Figures 6-1–6-3.

There was no statistically significant difference in mean IOP between the acetyl choline and control groups at baseline and at the end of surgery. However, the mean IOP for the control group was significantly greater than the acetyl choline group at 3, 6, 9, and 24 hours post surgery.

There was no significant difference in mean pupil size (horizontal and vertical) between the acetylcholine and control groups at baseline (undilated and dilated). At the end of surgery, the control group had a significantly greater mean pupil size (horizontal and vertical) than the acetyl choline group, and at 3 hours and at 24 hours. There was no difference in average pupil size between treatment groups at 6 and 9 hours post surgery.

The control group had a significantly greater mean pachymetry score at the start and end of surgery. However, there were no other significant pachymetry results.

An IOP spike was defined as a rise of 10 mmHg. from the measurement of IOP at baseline. Each patient was classified as either having or not having an IOP spike at 3, 6, 9, or 24 hours post surgery. In addition, patients were classified according to whether or not they had no spikes or at least one IOP spike during the course of the evaluation period (study overall). The Fisher's exact test was used to compare the proportion of patients with an IOP spike for each evaluation period. The results are listed in Table 6-2.

There were only 3 (15%) of the subjects in the acetylcholine group that had an IOP spike over the 24 hour post surgical period whereas there were 14 of 20 (70%) of the subjects in the control group that had an IOP spike. Furthermore, there was a significantly greater number of patients with IOP spikes in the control group as compared to the acetylcholine group at all follow up exam periods.

Table 6-1:   Mean and Standard Deviation for IOP, pupil size, and pachymetry by treatment group at each point of examination.

	Acetyl Choline		BSS Control	
IOP	mean	std	mean	std
start	16.55	3.02	14.86	2.85
3 hrs.	10.65	7.53	16.7	9.65
6 hrs.	16.00	8.16	23.70	9.93
9 hrs.	16.90	7.08	26.55	8.98
24 hrs.	19.05	5.10	23.38	8.76
Pupil				
start	6.63	0.96	6.00	1.10
end	3.11	1.05	5.36	1.01
3 hrs.	4.65	1.73	6.28	1.14
6 hrs.	5.98	1.50	6.43	1.23
9 hrs.	5.80	1.52	6.25	1.46
24 hrs.	3.95	0.76	4.62	1.37
Pachymetry				
start	0.554	0.041	0.581	0.039
end	0.590	0.053	0.625	0.045
3 hrs.	0.665	0.084	0.667	0.043
6 hrs.	0.667	0.067	0.638	0.048
9 hrs.	0.641	0.053	0.624	0.048
24hrs.	0.601	0.051	0.604	0.051

Discussion

Rich, Radtke, and Cohan were the first to document the pressure increases that occur within the initial 24 hours after cataract surgery.[5] In a series of uncomplicated intracapsular cataract extractions, they reported a maximum mean pressure rise of 21 mmHg. at a mean time of 6.8 hours after surgery. Of these patients, 75% of them had pressures greater than 30 mmHg. during the first 24 hours. Subsequent reports have confirmed similar findings, in association with intracapsular and extracapsular surgery, with and without the implantation of an intraocular lens.[3,4]

The cause of the increased intraocular pressure seen after cataract extraction is probably multifactorial in etiology. Decreased outflow facility appears to be the most significant factor. Rothkoff, Biedner, and Blumenthal found increased intraocular pressure (>24 mmHg.) in 14 of 60 patients (23%) who had intracapsular cataract extraction through a lim-

INTRAOCULAR PRESSURE

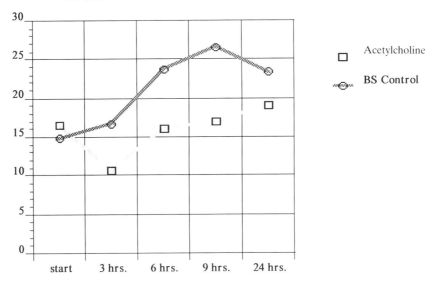

Figure 6-1:   Graphic display of intraocular pressure at each point of examination.

PUPIL DIAMETER

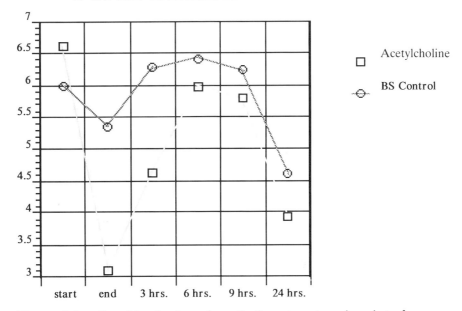

Figure 6-2:   Graphic display of pupil diameter at each point of examination.

PACHYMETRY

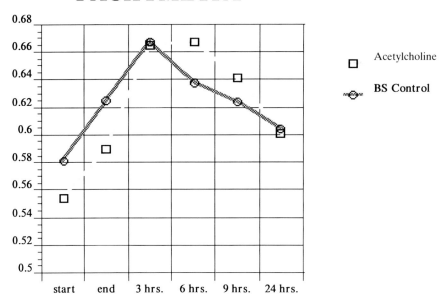

Figure 6-3: Graphic display of pachymetry at each point of examination.

bal incision vs. none of 34 patients who had a corneal cataract incision, implying that damage to the trabecular meshwork accounted for the decreased outflow facility.[24] Other studies have implicated permeability changes in the blood-aqueous barrier caused by postoperative inflammation and increased protein in the aqueous humor.[13,32] Tight wound closure also plays a role in increased postoperative pressure. Galin, Lin, and Obstbaum showed a positive correlation between the number of sutures placed and the rise in pressure at 24 hours.[16] The corneoscleral sutures themselves may contribute to increased pressure by distorting the angle or by increasing inflammation or localized corneal edema.

Table 6-2: Number of subjects with IOP spikes by treatment group and time of examination.

	End of Surgery	3 hrs.	6 hrs.	9 hrs.	24 hrs.	Study Overall
Acetyl Choline	0	0	2	2	2	3
Control	0	5	9	11	10	14
p-value	>.999	.021	.019	.004	.009	.001

The use of sodium hyaluronate during cataract surgery has been associated with transient increased postoperative intraocular pressure. The pressure rise peaks at two hours after injection, and returns to normal within 8 to 24 hours. Pressure increases were found to be significantly lower and less pronounced with anterior chamber washout of the sodium hyaluronate as opposed to leaving the sodium hyaluronate in the eye.

Sharp increases in intraocular pressure can be detrimental to susceptible eyes. Hayreh reported 13 cases of anterior ischemic optic neuropathy following cataract extraction.[19] Eleven of these patients had documented postoperative pressure increases. Patients with a history of postcataract ischemic optic neuropathy also have a higher risk of developing it in the second eye. Patients with preexisting glaucoma are also susceptible to a more intense short term pressure rise after cataract extraction Savage et al. found that 9.7% of glaucomatous eyes with severe preoperative field loss (split fixation or central field < 10 degrees) had additional field loss after extracapsular cataract extraction.[20] McGuigan et al. found a pressure rise of 7 mmHg. or greater in 62% of glaucomatous eyes compared to 10% of control eyes 24 hours after extracapsular cataract extraction.[21]

Acetylcholine is the naturally occurring neurohumoral transmitter for autonomic ganglia and skeletal muscle (nicotinic action) and for postganglionic parasympathetic nerve fibers (muscarinic action). It is a natural vasodilator, a cardiac depressant, and a stimulant of the vagus nerve and the entire parasympathetic nervous system. The muscarinic actions can be abolished by atropine while the nicotinic actions are blocked by tubocurarine.[33] Acetylcholine in high doses produces coronary vasodilation, decreased myocardial contractility, and bradycardia.[34] Continuous doses of acetylcholine cause cardiac arrest.[35]

In the eye, postganglionic parasympathetic fibers from the ciliary ganglion innervate the sphincter pupillae, causing miosis, and the ciliary muscle, resulting in changes in accommodation and in the facility of outflow. Exogenous acetylcholine administered intracamerally can duplicate some of the effects of parasympathetic stimulation. Amsler and Verrey first established the miotic effect of intracameral acetylcholine in 1949.[36] Barraquer may have been the first to use acetylcholine routinely in anterior segment surgery.[37] Since then the value of acetylcholine induced miosis has been established for cataract surgery and intraocular lens implantation.[38-44] Acetylcholine has also been used in cases of acute retinal vascular occlusion as a retrobulbar injection to achieve vasodilation of the retinal and choroidal blood vessels.[45]

As with other cholinergic agents, pharmacologic preparations of acetylcholine have been shown to have a direct effect on ciliary muscle preparations,[46] which would be expected to increase outflow facility through effects of the trabecular meshwork. Additionally, acetylcholine appears to have an inhibitory effect on aqueous secretion.[47] The combination of these two factors results in a drop in intraocular pressure.

Acetylcholine is rapidly broken down by the action of acetylcholinesterase. Thus it is commonly classified as a short acting miotic.

Carbachol (carbaminoylcholine) is a potent synthetic choline ester, differing from acetylcholine by a carbaminoyl (NH_2CO) group in place of an acetyl (CH_3CO) group attached to the choline base. Its general pharmacologic properties were first described by Kreitmair in 1932.[48] Like acetylcholine, carbachol is primarily a direct-acting agent,[49] with muscarinic and nicotinic effects. It may also cause the release of endogenous acetylcholine from cholinergic nerve fiber terminals[50] or partially inhibit cholinesterase. It has an inhibitory effect on secretion by the ciliary body. Because carbachol is resistant to hydrolysis by cholinesterase, it is active for much longer than acetylcholine. On a weight for weight basis, it is 100 times more potent than acetylcholine.[51] Thus commercial preparations are a 0.01% solution compared to 1.0% for acetylcholine.

Topical carbachol has been used as an anti-glaucoma medication for over 50 years.[52] Because the molecule carries a positive charge, it penetrates poorly through the corneal epithelium. Surfactants such as benzalkonium chloride are necessary to increase corneal penetration. In 1965, Reed described the use of intracameral carbachol as an alternative to acetylcholine for intraocular miosis.[53] Subsequent clinical and experimental studies have established that the miotic effect of carbachol is more intense and of longer duration than with acetylcholine.[42,54,55]

Systemic effects from intraocular use of acetylcholine are rare. Those reported include hypotension, bradycardia, bronchospasm, and sweating. Systemic effects from carbachol are clinically more common, with patients complaining of brow ache, headache, nausea, abdominal cramps and tightness in the urinary bladder. Corneal clouding, persistent bullous keratopathy and post operative iritis following cataract extraction with utilization of intraocular carbachol have been occasionally reported.[59,60]

Hollands, Drance, and Schulzer studied a group of patients, 3, 6, 9, and 24 hours after they received either acetylcholine or balanced salt control during cataract extraction without the use of a viscoelastic. They reported that whereas the control group had elevated intraocular pressure throughout the first 24 hours, the acetylcholine group was normotensive, with intraocular pressures similar to baseline. The difference between the acetylcholine group and the controls was significant at 3 and 6 hours, while the similarity of the acetylcholine group to baseline was significant at all measurements.[1]

Hollands, Drance, and Schulzer then repeated the exact study, this time comparing patients who received carbachol during cataract surgery to those receiving BSS controls. This time the carbachol group was not normotensive, but lower than baseline for intraocular pressure. This hypotensive effect lasted throughout the postoperative period. The control group was again hypertensive. The differences were significant at all measurements.[2]

A subsequent study by Linn et al. further emphasized the hypotensive effect of carbachol. After a 0.5 ml injection into the anterior chamber at the close of cataract surgery with viscoelastic, the mean intraocular pressure throughout the first 48 hours was less than 10 mmHg., with the mean at 48 hours of only 4.2 mmHg.[28]

Our study confirmed that of Hollands, Drance,and Schulzer, though differing in protocol since all our patients received hyaluronate visco-elastic while their study was done without viscoelastics. Whereas their study demonstrated the efficacy of acetylcholine in control of intraocular pressure in cataract surgery without viscoelastic, ours showed that acetyl choline was equally effective in surgery with the use of viscoelastic.

Thus both acetylcholine and carbachol have been shown to prevent postoperative elevations in intraocular pressure, acetylcholine by maintaining the intraocular pressure in a normotensive range, carbachol by lowering pressure to a hypotensive or even hypotonous extent.

In the normal eye, the elasticity and muscular tone of the choroid creates a negative pressure in the suprachoroidal space and attracts fluid from the anterior chamber. A pressure gradient exists between the aqueous and vitreous cavities and the suprachoroidal space. The lower pressure within the suprachoroidal space acts to push the choroid outward, holding it against the inner surface of the sclera.[61]

When the intraocular pressure is severely reduced, the venous pressure inside the eye becomes greater than the intraocular pressure and the Starling equilibrium shifts towards extravascular fluid accumulation. In addition, hypotony causes the pressure gradient across the sclera to diminish and thus the rate of loss of fluid through the sclera diminishes as well. If the rate of loss becomes smaller than the rate of entry, fluid will accumulate in the suprachoroidal space and spontaneous detachment of the choroid will occur. If the colloid concentration in the suprachoroidal space rises due to decreased bulk outflow through the sclera, the colloid osmotic absorptive forces of the plasma are reduced and fluid accumulation in the suprachoroidal space will be more rapid. Inflammation accelerates this process because of the greater rate of movement of colloids into the suprachoroidal fluid. Combined with hypotony, inflammation produces a rapid accumulation of fluid in the suprachoroidal space and a resultant choroidal detachment.[61]

Pathologic studies of human enucleated eyes with acute hypotony show massive edematous dilatation of the uvea, especially the pars plicata of the ciliary body. The posterior choroid is diffusely thickened and peripheral choroidal detachments are seen. The increased volume of the choroid leads to folds of Bruch's membrane and the retina. Retinal signs are cystoid degeneration, especially in the area of the outer plexiform layer and inner nuclear layer, and wrinkling of the inner limiting membrane.[62]

The true incidence of choroidal detachment in the early postoperative period after cataract surgery is unknown. Several studies have reported incidences of 2.6% to 10% for clinically detectable choroidal detachments, while many more have subclinical detachments.[63] Fortunately, resolution is usually associated with rapid normalization of the intraocular pressure and reduction of intraocular inflammation.

Although the permanent ocular effects of short term hypotony are not known, the most likely effects will occur in the retina where leakage of intravascular fluid will occur due to instability of fine capillaries. Potentially, this could lead to a higher incidence of cystoid macular edema.

Another factor related to the use of miotics that might have an effect on cystoid macular edema is the effect on intraocular inflammation from prolonged miosis. Delay in the reestablishment of the blood aqueous barrier may lead to increased levels of aqueous protein as well as higher levels of intraocular prostaglandins.

The Kowa FC-1000 is a diagnostic instrument to objectively measure the amount of protein (flare) and the number of white blood cells (cells) in the anterior chamber. With this instrument, not only can reproducible measurements made at each time interval, but in addition, changes in the amount of inflammation over time can be monitored.

In a separate study, patients undergoing cataract extraction were randomly assigned to receive either acetylcholine solution, carbachol solution, or balanced salt solution controls twice during cataract surgery, once immediately after placement of the posterior chamber intraocular lens, and then at the very end of the surgery. The surgical procedure and inclusion and exclusion criteria were the same as in our study of IOP. Measurements of cell and flare were made on the first and eighth postoperative days by the same technician. Patients received no steroids at the time of surgery either topically or subconjunctivally, and were begun on a suspension of prednisolone acetate 1% four times a day beginning after their measurement on the first postoperative day.

The preliminary data for this study is shown in Table 6-3 and in Figures 6-4 and 6-5. The measurement of both flare and cell are statistically similar for the control group and the acetylcholine group at both the first and the eighth postoperative day. The measurements for the carbachol group are significantly higher for both cell and flare than the acetylcholine or control groups at both the first and eighth postoperative day.

We presume that it is the prolonged intense miosis associated with carbachol that is responsible for the prolonged inflammation that we measure. Even though the effect on the pupil is no longer present on the eighth postoperative day, increased levels of inflammation can still be measured due to the delay in reestablishment of the blood aqueous barrier.

Table 6-3:   Cell and flare measurements.

DRUG	CELL	FLARE
Miostat		
1 day	41.4	98.08
1 week	9.98	42.31
Miochol		
1 day	27.13	34.40
1 week	3.27	19.89
BS Control		
1 day	30.06	42.80
1 week	3.65	19.50

INFLAMMATION - Cell

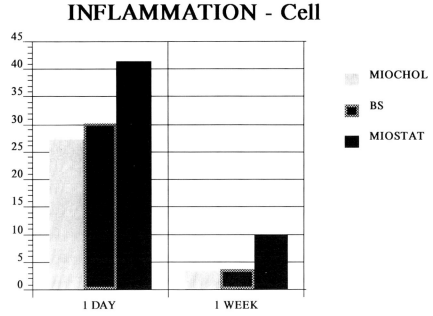

Figure 6-4:   Graphic display of inflammation-cell.

INFLAMMATION - Flare

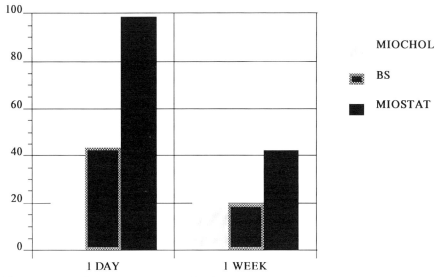

Figure 6-5:   Graphic display of inflammation-flare.

The clinical significance of prolonged inflammation needs to be determined. One argument against the use of a long acting miotic has been the clinical impression that there is more pigment deposition on the surface of intraocular lenses when such a miotic is used.[18] More significant would be a delay in visual recovery due to prolonged inflammation and the resultant development of cystoid macular edema. It would be interesting to compare angiographically the rate of development of cystoid macular edema among patients receiving acetylcholine to those receiving carbachol during their cataract surgery.

The cataract surgeon needs to weigh the benefit versus the risk in the use of these drugs. In one of my other chapters in this book I present the results of experiments that showed toxicity to the corneal endothelium from carbachol and not from acetylcholine. The hypotonous changes in the choroid and retina along with the corneal endothelial toxicity and prolonged post-operative inflammation suggest that carbachol not be used routinely in cataract surgery.

When I was a resident, I asked by attending why it was that aphakic eyes tend to have paler optic nerves than do phakic eyes. I was told that it was an optical artifact caused by the absence of the crystalline lens. I did not accept that answer then as I do not now. In clinical practice, the intraocular pressure is not usually measured until the first postoperative day, and it is apparent from these and other studies that in many patients, there will be a significant increase in intraocular pressure that will escape detection. Though most patients will not develop clinically significant visual changes as a result of this pressure spike, the potential exists for permanent ischemic optic nerve head damage, especially in individuals with preexisting vascular insufficiency. Hayreh described 13 cases of anterior ischemic optic neuropathy that developed immediately after uncomplicated cataract surgery, and concluded that the ischemic damage was due to a drop in the capillary perfusion pressure, resulting from an increase in intraocular pressure in eyes already suffering from compromised optic nerve circulation. In addition, patients who developed optic nerve ischemia after cataract surgery were more likely to develop the same condition in the fellow eye.[19]

My recommendation as a result of the two studies presented in this manuscript would be to use acetylcholine, a short acting miotic for routine patients without a history of glaucoma or other tendency towards elevated intraocular pressure. Acetylcholine has been shown to maintain intraocular pressure within a normal range during the first 24 hours after surgery and blunts the IOP spike that would otherwise occur. Acetylcholine does not increase intraocular inflammation nor, as it is naturally occurring in the anterior chamber, is it toxic to the endothelium. Carbachol, a long acting miotic with a more intense and prolonged effect on both miosis and intraocular pressure, should be reserved for those patients with glaucoma, for whom any pressure elevation might have a disastrous effect on the optic nerve. For these patients, the benefit of intraocular pressure control more than outweighs the risk from an increase in postoperative inflammation.

For all patients, our goal should be normotensive eyes with minimum postoperative inflammation. By tailoring our choice of agents to the particular needs of our patients, we should be able to achieve this objective.

References

1. Hollands MH, Drance SM, Schulzer M: The effect of acetylcholine on early postoperative intraocular pressure. Am J Ophthalmol, 1987, 103:749–53.
2. Hollands MH, Drance SM, Schulzer M: The effect of intracameral carbachol on intraocular pressure after cataract extraction. Am J Ophthalmol, 1987, 104:225–8.
3. Naeser K, Thin K, Hansen TE et al.: Intraocular pressure in the first days after implantation of posterior chamber lenses with the use of sodium hyaluronate (Healon). Acta Ophthalmologica, 1986, 64:330–7.
4. Haimann MH, Phelps CD: Prophylactic timolol for the prevention of high intraocular pressure after cataract extraction. Ophthalmology, 1981, 88:233–8.
5. Rich WJ, Radke ND, Cohan BE: Early ocular hypertension after cataract extraction. Br J Ophthalmol, 1974, 58:725–31.
6. Sheppard DD, Kiolker AE, Hoskins HD et al.: IOP greater than 33 mm Hg. in postoperative extracapsular cataract-posterior chamber intraocular lens patients. J Cataract Refract Surg, 1987, 13:568–573.
7. Gormaz A: Ocular tension after cataract surgery. Am J Ophthalmol, 1962, 53:832.
8. Kirsch RE: Glaucoma following cataract extraction associated with use of alpha-chymotrypsin. Arch Ophthalmol, 1964, 72:612.
9. Galin MA, Barasch KR, Harris: Enzymatic zonulolysis and intraocular pressure. Am J Ophthalmol, 1966, 61:690.
10. Rich WJ: Intraocular pressure and wound closure after cataract extraction. Trans Ophthalmol Soc U.K. 1968, 88:437.
11. Cherfan GM, Rich WJ, Wright G: Raised intraocular pressure and other problems with sodium hyaluronate and cataract surgery. Trans Ophthalmol Soc U.K. 1983, 103:277.
12. Brown SV, Tye JG, McPherson SD: Intraocular pressure after intracapsular cataract extraction. Ophthalmic Surg., 1984, 15:389.
13. Rich WJ. Further studies on early postoperative ocular hypertension following cataract extraction. Trans Ophthalmol Soc U.K., 1969, 89:639.
14. Packer AJ, Fraioli AJ, Epstein DL: The effect of timolol and acetazolamide on transient intraocular pressure elevation following cataract extraction with alphachymotrypsin. Ophthalmology, 1981, 88:239.
15. Tomoda T, Tuberville AW, Wood TO: Timolol and postoperative intraocular pressure. Am Intraocular Implant Soc J, 1984, 10:180.
16. Galin MA, Lin LL, Obstbaum SA: Cataract extraction and intraocular pressure. Trans Ophthalmol Soc U.K., 1978, 98:124.

5555

555555

17. Tuberville AW, Tomoda T, Nissenkorn I, Wood TO: Post surgical intraocular pressure elevation. Am Intraocular Implant Soc J. 1983, 9:309.
18. Sanders DR, ed., IOP after cataract surgery. Ocular Surgery News, supplement to April 1, 1988 issue, p. 8.
19. Hayreh SS: Anterior ischemic optic neuropathy IV. Occurrence after cataract surgery. Arch Ophthalmol, 1980, 98:1410.
20. Savage JA, Thomas JV, Belcher CD, Simmons RJ: Extracapsular cataract extraction and posterior chamber intraocular lens implantation in glaucomatous eyes. Ophthalmology, 1985, 92:1506.
21. McGuigan LJ, Gottsch J, Stark WJ, Maumenee AE, Guigley HA: Extracapsular cataract extraction and posterior chamber lens implantation in eyes with preexisting glaucoma, Arch Ophthalmol, 1986, 104:1301.
22. Passo MS, Ernest JT, Goldstick TK: Hyaluronate increases intraocular pressure when used in cataract extraction. Br J Ophthalmol, 1985, 69:572–5.
23. Olivius E, Thorburn W: Intraocular pressure after cataract surgery with Healon. Am Intra-Ocular Implant Soc J. 1985, 11:480–2.
24. Rothkoff L, Biedner B, Blumenthal M: The effect of corneal section on early increased intraocular pressure after cataract extraction. Am J Ophthalmol, 1978, 85:337.
25. Biedner BZ, Rosenblatt I, David R, Sacks U: The effect of timolol on early increased intraocular pressure after cataract extraction. Glaucoma, 1982, 4:53.
26. West DR, Lischwe TD, Thompson VM, Ide CH: Comparative efficacy of the B-blockers for the prevention of increased intraocular pressure after cataract extraction, Am J Ophthalmol, 1988, 106:168.
27. Ruiz RS, Wilson CA, Musgrove KH, Prager TC: Management of increased intraocular pressure after cataract surgery. Am J Ophthalmol, 1987, 103:487.
28. Linn DK, Zimmerman TJ, Nardin GF et al.: Effect of Intracameral carbachol on intraocular pressure after cataract extraction. Am J Ophthalmol, 1989, 107:133–6.
29. Ruiz RS, Rhem NM, Prager TC: Effects of carbachol and acetylcholine on intraocular pressure after cataract extraction. Am J Ophthalmol, 1989, 107:7.
30. McKenzie JW, Boggs MB: Comparison of postoperative intraocular pressures after use of Miochol and Miostat. J Cataract Refract Surg, 1989, 15:185.
31. Zimmerman TJ, Wheeler TM: Miotics:side effects and ways to avoid them. Ophthalmology, 1982, 89:76.
32. Sears D, Sears M: Blood-aqueous barrier and alpha chymotrypsin glaucoma in rabbits. Am J Ophthalmol, 1974, 77:378.
33. Gombos DS: Acetylcholine in Ophthalmology: a revisit. Ann Ophthalmol. 1988, 20:455.
34. Blumenthal MR, Wang H, Markee S et al.: Effects of acetylcholine on the heart. J Physiol (Lond), 1968, 8:1280.

35. Rook AR: Acetylcholine-induced cardiac arrest during cerebrovascular surgery: A clinical trial. J Am Optom Assoc, 1973, 73:287.

36. Amsler M, Verrey F: Mydriase et myose directes en instances par les mediateurs chimiques. Ann Ocul, 1949, 182:936.

37. Barraquer JI: Acetylcholine as a miotic agent for use in surgery. Am J Ophthalmol, 1964, 57:406.

38. Harley RD, Mishler JE: Acetylcholine in cataract surgery. Am J Ophthalmol, 1964, 57:817.

39. Harley RD, Mishler JE: Acetylcholine in cataract surgery. Br J Ophthalmol, 1966, 50:429.

40. Ray RR: Use of acetylcholine in peripheral iridectomy. Am J Ophthalmol, 1965, 60:728.

41. Rizzuti AB: Acetylcholine in surgery of the lens, iris and cornea. Am J Ophthalmol, 1967, 63:484.

42. Beasley H: Miotics in cataract surgery. Arch Ophthalmol, 1972, 88:49.

43. Douglas GR: A comparison of acetylcholine and carbachol following cataract extraction. Can J Ophthalmol, 1973, 8:75.

44. Schirmer RA: Intraocular instillation of acetylcholine in anterior segment operations. Eye Ear Nose Throat J, 1966, 28:63.

45. Gombos GM: Retinal vascular occlusions and their treatment with low molecular weight dextrans and vasodilators: Report of six years experience. Ann Ophthalmol, 1978, 10:579.

46. van Alphen GW, Robinette SL, Macri FJ: Drug effects on ciliary muscle and choroid preparations in vitro. Arch Ophthalmol, 1962, 68:81.

47. Berggren L: Effect of parasympathomimetic and sympathomimetic drugs on secretion in vitro by the ciliary processes of the rabbit eye. Invest Ophthalmol, 1965, 4:91.

48. Kreitmair H: Eine neue Klasse cholinester, Arch Exp. Pathol Pharmakol, 1932, 164:346.

49. Yamauchi LD, Patil PN: Relative potency of cholinomimetic drugs on the bovine iris sphincter strips. Invest Ophthalmol, 1973, 12:80.

50. McKinstry DN, Koelle GB: Effects of drugs on acetylcholine release from the cat superior cervical ganglion by carbachol and by preganglionic stimulation. J Pharmacol Exp Ther, 1967, 157:328.

51. McDonald TO, Beasley G, Borgann A et al.: Intraocular administration of carbamylcholine chloride. Ann Ophthalmol. 1969, 1:232.

52. O'Brien CS, Swan KC: Carbaminoylcholine chloride in the treatment of glaucoma simplex. Arch Ophthalmol, 1942, 27:253.

53. Reed H: Use of carbamylcholine chloride. Am J Ophthalmol, 1965, 59:955.

54. Beasley H, Borgmann AR, McDonald TO, Belluscio PR: Carbachol in cataract surgery. Arch Ophthalmol, 1968, 80:39.

55. Douglas G: A comparison of acetylcholine and carbachol following cataract extraction. Can J Ophthalmol, 1973, 8:75.

56. Babinski M, Smith B, Wickerham EP: Hypotension and bradycardia following intraocular acetylcholine injection. Arch Ophthalmol, 1976, 94:675.

57. Gombos GM: Systemic reactions following intraocular acetylcholine instillation. Ann Ophthalmol, 1982, 14:592.
58. Brinkley JR, Henrick A: Vascular hypotension and bradycardia following intraocular injection of acetylcholine during cataract surgery. Am J Ophthalmol, 1984, 97:40.
59. Physicians' Desk Reference For Ophthalmology, Oradell, N.J., Medical Economics Co., 17th edition, 1989, p. 83.
60. McDonald TO, Roberts MD, Borgmann AR: Intraocular safety of carbamylcholine chloride in rabbit eyes. Ann Ophthalmol, 1970, 2:878.
61. Brubaker RF, Peterson JE: Ciliochoroidal detachment. Survey of Ophthalmol, 1983, 27(5):281–8.
62. Volcker HE, Naumann GOH: Morphology of uveal and retinal edemas in acute and persisting hypotony. Mod. Probl. Ophthal., 1979, 20:34–41.
63. Shah RR: Flat anterior chamber and choroidal detachment in aphakia. Brit J Ophthalmol, 1971, 55:48.

Chapter 7

POSTERIOR SEGMENT COMPLICATIONS IN CATARACT AND LENS IMPLANT SURGERY

Hal D. Balyeat, MD

Recently, Stark et al. reported on trends in intraocular lens implantation.[1] According to reports form IOL manufacturers to the FDA, 1,174,000 IOLs were implanted in the United States during a 12–month period ending January 1989. Ninety-three percent of these lenses were posterior chamber lenses and 7% were anterior chamber lenses. In 1983, 495,000 intraocular lenses were implanted in the United States. This means that the number of implant cases more than doubled during a 6 year period. The authors correctly point out that the rise was related to a number of factors, among them the increasing skill in IOL surgery, an increasing acceptance of implantation by patients, and a growing appreciation by the public and ophthalmologists that the improved rehabilitation provided by pseudophakia over aphakia justified a change in the indications for surgery. Interestingly, when an adjustment is made for an average of 2% annual increase in the number of people 65 years of age and older, there has been a relative decline in the number of intraocular lenses implanted during the last three six–month periods ending January 1989. These figures seem to indicate a definite slowing in the number of cataract extractions performed annually in the United States. Cataract surgery, regardless of the method employed, increases the risk of subsequent retinal detachment. Norton, speaking at the Second Cataract Congress in 1971 stated, "So long as you cataract surgeons keep taking them out, we retinal surgeons will never go out of business."[2]

Retinal Detachment

What is the incidence of retinal detachment following cataract surgery? Retinal detachment develops approximately 0.005 to 0.010% of phakic individuals annually (5–10 per 100,000 population).[3] In phakic myopes the incidence rises to at least 1% with rates increasing as the degree of myopia increases. Intraocular surgery, specifically cataract extraction, is a major contributing factor to retinal detachment. Approximately 3% of the adult population has had cataract surgery, but as many as 40% of retinal detachments occur in aphakic or pseudophakic eyes.[4] The increased incidence of retinal detachment after uncomplicated cataract extraction is due to changes in the vitreous gel leading to vitreoretinal traction. The incidence of posterior vitreous detachment increases significantly following cataract extraction.

In a study of 201 autopsy eyes,[5] 146 cases had prior intracapsular cataract extraction with an incidence of posterior vitreous detachment of 84%. Twenty-five eyes had extracapsular surgery with a posterior capsulotomy, and the incidence of posterior vitreous detachment was 76%. The incidence of posterior vitreous detachment in 30 eyes with an intact posterior capsule was 40%. Prior to extracapsular cataract surgery and intraocular lens implantation the increased incidence of posterior vitreous detachment was thought to be due in part to the mechanical displacement of the anterior vitreous through the pupillary aperature into the anterior chamber. However, detectable anterior vitreous changes are unusual after extracapsular cataract extraction and although rupture of the anterior vitreous surface may occur after capsulotomy, forward displacement of the vitreous is usually prevented by the implant. Osterlin has measured the concentration of hyaluronic acid in both human subjects and laboratory animals after intracapsular and extracapsular surgery and has found a measurable reduction in hyaluronic acid content in the vitreous cavity when compared to fellow phakic eyes.[6,7,8] In the owl monkey, he found a measurable reduction in hyaluronic acid content occurred within one week after intracapsular extraction while the concentration remained unchanged in eyes with an intact posterior capsule when evaluated four weeks postoperatively. Hyaluronic acid loss results in less stability of the collagen fibrils resulting in increasing amounts of fluid vitreous.

Retinal tears occur in approximately 10% to 15% of cases at the time of posterior vitreous detachment.[9] This incidence is apparently the same for phakic as well as aphakic eyes. Hovland[10] studied 100 aphakic eyes of individuals with aphakic retinal detachment in the fellow eye. Posterior vitreous detachment was present in 60 of the fellow eyes. Retinal tears were found in 17(28%) of these 60 eyes. One of the 60 eyes with a previously documented posterior vitreous separation subsequently developed a new retinal tear. Of the remaining 40 eyes, 11 (28%) developed posterior vitreous detachments with retinal tears occurring in 8 (73%) of these cases.

These data indicate that the presence of a posterior vitreous detachment in a non-myopic eye prior to cataract surgery lessens the chance of a retinal detachment occurring postoperatively. The problem, of course, is determining whether or not a posterior vitreous detachment has occurred preoperatively. An optically empty vitreous and/or a well-defined posterior vitreous surface does not insure the presence of a posterior vitreous detachment. Only by demonstrating the presence of a fibrotic annulus on the posterior vitreous surface can one be sure of the diagnosis. If a posterior vitreous detachment can be documented clinically prior to cataract extraction in a non-myopic eye, the incidence of postoperative retinal detachment following uncomplicated cataract extraction with an intact posterior capsule should be less than 1%. We are currently studying the incidence of posterior vitreous detachment in eyes of patients undergoing extracapsular cataract extraction with posterior chamber lens implantation.

Factors which increase the incidence of retinal detachment following cataract surgery are: 1) preoperative (high myopia, previous history of retinal detachment in the fellow eye, family history of retinal detachment, lattice degeneration, relative youth, male sex); 2) intraoperative (primary discission and vitreous loss); and 3) postoperative (posterior capsulotomy).

Historically, the most frequent association with the development of aphakic retinal detachment has been myopia with retinal detachment occurring in 40% of myopic eyes greater than ten diopters.[11] In extracapsular pseudophakic eyes the incidence is considerably lower, but nonetheless significantly higher than in the non-high-myope population, although two studies noted a relatively low incidence of retinal detachment in myopes.[12,13] These studies defined myopia based on postoperative refraction or IOL power rather than axial length. In a series of 3065 consecutive cases of extracapsular cataract extraction with posterior chamber lens implant Smith et al.[14] found the incidence of retinal detachment to be 1.7% in a group of eyes followed for at least one year. The incidence of retinal detachment in the group of moderate myopes (axial length $> 25 < 26.5$ mm) was 6.3%. Surprisingly, this incidence was greater than in a group of highly myopic eyes (axial length > 26.5 mm) 4.8%. Nonetheless, these figures represent a four and three-fold increase when compared to a control group of non-myopic eyes. Lindstrom, reporting in the 1988 Transactions of the New Orleans Academy of Ophthalmology[15] found an incidence of 7.04% retinal detachment rate (5/71) in axial myopes (25.00 mm>). The mean axial length for the five eyes with retinal detachment was 28.60 mm, compared to an overall mean axial length of 27.18 mm for the entire myopic group. Four of the five eyes that developed a retinal detachment had received a posterior chamber lens implant. The presence or absence of implants did not seem to affect the incidence of retinal detachment. None of the eyes in the study underwent inadvertent posterior capsule rupture or primary capsulotomy at the time of surgery. Sixty-three of the 71 axially myopic eyes maintained an intact posterior capsule throughout the course of the study. Three of the 63 myopic eyes (4.76%) with an intact posterior capsule went on to develop retinal detachment. Eight of the 71 myopic eyes underwent a YAG capsulotomy with 2 (25%) of these eyes developing a retinal detachment.

Patients with a history of retinal detachment in the fellow eye may have a four fold increase in the risk of retinal detachment compared to eyes that remain phakic.[16] In a study by Coonan et al.[17] patients with myopia in excess of 8 diopters developed retinal detachment with a frequency of 3.5% (3/86). The incidence of retinal detachment in patients with a previous detachment in the fellow eye was 5.9% (4/68).

Lattice degeneration occurs in about 8% of eyes in the general population, but it is present in 20% to 30% of retinal detachment cases. Lattice degeneration, however, is a rare cause of retinal detachment in phakic patients without other predisposing factors. Byer observed 204 untreated patients with lattice degeneration for 3 to 10 years without the occurrence of a single case of retinal detachment.[18] The incidence of lattice degeneration is the same in the phakic and psuedophakic population, but there is a lower incidence of lattice degeneration in pseudophakic detachments compared to phakic detachments. There is a higher incidence of lattice degeneration in myopic eyes compared to non-myopes.

Vitreous loss at the time of surgery has been indited as a predisposition to retinal detachment. Wilkinson reported an incidence of vitreous loss of 4.2% in a series of 1500 eyes undergoing phacoemulsification.[19] Fourteen percent of these patients developed retinal detachment. Other series report an incidence of retinal detachment following vitreous loss of 6.8 to 15.4%.[20,21]

In summary, a myope with an axial length 25.00 mm or greater may have a 5–7% chance of developing a retinal detachment following uneventful extracapsular cataract extraction with an intact posterior capsule. Retention of an intact posterior capsule reduces the incidence of retinal detachment in axial myopes but the presence of myopia raises the postoperative rate of retinal detachment dramatically. The higher the myopia, the higher the retinal detachment rate.

What is the risk of retinal detachment following Nd-YAG posterior capsulotomy? Koch, et al. retrospectively studied 121 eyes followed at least one year after YAG laser capsulotomy.[22] Retinal complications occurred in 3 (2.5%) of these eyes and in 2 (3.6%) of 55 eyes followed for 2 years. There were four retinal detachment and one symptomatic retinal tear. No cases of clinical cystoid macular edema were noted. The five eyes with retinal complications had a mean axial length of 25.3 mm. There were no retinal complications in eyes with axial lengths of 24 mm or less. The incidence of retinal detachment in eyes of axial length 25 mm or greater was 10%. The incidence of retinal complications in patients under age 60 with axial lengths greater than 24 mm was 9%. Males with axial lengths greater than 24 mm had a retinal complication of 17%.

In a study of 25 eyes in 24 patients with retinal detachment after YAG laser posterior capsulotomy, Leff et al.[23] found that four patients had a history of retinal detachment in the fellow eye, two had preoperative high myopia, and two had lattice degeneration. This means that approximately one-third of the study eyes exhibited a preoperative risk factor for retinal detachment.

In another retrospective review of consecutive eyes that had undergone YAG laser posterior capsulotomy and had been followed for a minimum of three months, 13 (3.6%) eyes developed retinal detachment.[24] Ten of these eyes had posterior chamber lenses and three eyes were aphakic. The incidence of retinal detachment in the posterior chamber lens subgroup was 3.6% and 4.2% in the aphakic group. The incidence of retinal detachment in the posterior chamber lens subgroup in eyes with axial length greater than 25.00 mm was 8.3%. In male axial myopes the incidence was 17.6%. There was a 9.6% incidence of retinal detachment in the group of patients who had one or more of the three risk factors (axial myopia $\geq$ 25.00 mm, lattice degeneration, or previous retinal detachment in the fellow eye).

A study by Ober, et al.[25] failed to demonstrate a relationship between capsulotomy size, laser energy required to create the capsulotomy and retinal detachment.

In summary, a non-myope without risk factors has a relatively small chance of having a retinal detachment following YAG capsulotomy; not significantly different than his chance of detachment following uneventful cataract surgery. However, axial myopes have a 8–10% chance of retinal detachment following YAG capsulotomy and the addition of other risk factors (male gender, youth, lattice degeneration, previous retinal detachment in the fellow eye) increases the chances of retinal detachment significantly. A young male myope has an approximate 17% chance of experiencing a retinal detachment.[22,24] These figures are relatively conservative since most studies have limited follow-up of two years or less. Although annual rates will decrease after two years, one may anticipate an increase in the percentage of retinal detachments occurring after cataract extraction and YAG capsulotomy.

Cystoid Macular Edema

Cystoid macular edema (CME) remains an important cause of disappointing postoperative visual acuity. Fortunately, the incidence of persistent visually significant CME is relatively low. Bradford et al. retrospectively reviewed 20 psuedophakic eyes with posterior chamber lenses and clinical CME.[26] Resolution of the symptomatic clinical CME was observed in 18 (90%) of the 20 eyes. Clearing occurred within the first 12 months in 14 eyes (78%) and within 24 months in 17 (94%). Six of the seven eyes (86%) with a primary posterior capsulotomy experienced resolution of the CME as did 12 (92%) of the 13 eyes with an intact capsule. Stark et al. studied 961 eyes undergoing planned extracapsular surgery with posterior chamber lens implantation.[27] Follow-up ranged from 3 to 44 months with an average of 19 months. Clinical cystoid macular edema was defined as a reduction in prior distance and/or near visual acuity of one line or more on the Snellen chart, associated with ophthalmoscopically visible cystoid changes in the macula or fluorescein angiographic evidence of CME. The incidence of clinical CME in their series was 2.0%. The median time of onset was 8 weeks (range, 2–64). In 95% of cases, the onset of CME was less than 28 weeks. There were 17 cases of transient CME and 3 cases of persistent CME. Eighty-five percent of eyes with CME had a posterior capsulotomy while 81% of all patients had a capsulotomy at the time of surgery. It was the opinion of the authors that if clinically significant persistent CME developed in only 0.3% of uncomplicated cases, then any modification of technique that had a favorable treatment effect in 50%

of cases would require a study of about 25,000 cases to demonstrate statistical significance.

Jaffe et al. studied angiographic and clinical CME in patients undergoing both intracapsular and extracapsular cataract extraction with and without intraocular lens implantation.[28] In uncomplicated cases of ECCE with posterior chamber lens and primary capsulotomy, the incidence of angiographic CME was 2.9% (3/103) and the incidence of clinical CME was 0.0%. After complicated surgery (vitreous loss, capsule rupture, zonular dialysis) the incidence of angiographic CME was 29.5% (18/61) with 18% (11/61) exhibiting clinical CME. Does a primary capsulotomy increase the incidence of angiographic and/or clinical CME? In one study, 288 patients were randomly assigned to capsulotomy or non-capsulotomy following uneventful ECCE and posterior chamber lens implantations.[29] Fluorescein angiograms were performed in 63% of the cases. Angiographic CME was noted in 21.5% (20/93) of primary capsulotomy eyes and 5.5% (4/71) of intact capsule eyes. It was the author's conclusion that the presence of an intact capsule at the time of surgery significantly decreased the angiographic incidence of CME and that the CME in the intact capsule group was milder.

In an attempt to further examine the incidence of angiographic CME occurring six weeks and six months after posterior chamber IOL implantation as a function of the status of the posterior capsule we performed a prospective study of 162 eyes of which 141 were randomized into either a primary capsulotomy or a capsule-intact group.[30] The eyes which were not randomized due to intraoperative surgical complications were included in the follow-up studies. Angiograms were obtained in 96% of the cases. Angiographic CME was observed in 24% of the capsulotomy group and 16% of the capsule intact group.

Fluorescein leakage was observed in only 11% of the nonrandomized (complicated surgery) group. Two patients (3%) of cases with capsulotomies exhibited clinical CME at six weeks and 1 case (1%) of the intact-capsule group demonstrated clinical CME. A subgroup of 100 randomized cases and 20 nonrandomized cases were studied angiographically at six months. An abnormal angiogram was recorded in 2 (4%) cases in each of the intact-capsule and capsulotomy cases. No CME was observed in the nonrandomized cases. Two patients (4%) of the capsulotomy cases had clinical CME at six months. Clinical CME was not observed in the capsule intact or in the nonrandomized series. Clinical CME was unusual in this series. It was present six weeks after surgery in 3 (2.1%) of 141 randomized cases and in (4.5%) of 21 nonrandomized cases. Clinical CME was present in 2 (1.7%) of cases six months after surgery and in both instances it occurred in association with an open capsule. Unfortunately, as pointed out by Javitt, this study was flawed by an inadequate study population.[31] This involves the concept of power of a study which is defined as the likelihood that a statistically significant difference will be detected if it exists. The power of a study is determined by an interaction of the magnitude of the outcome variable, the magnitude of the expected difference between groups, and the size of the study population. Javitt noted that to have 80% power in detecting a statistically significant 33% relative decrease in the rate of CME would require a sample size of 390 patients in both capsulotomy and capsule-intact groups. In spite of these shortcomings and despite the absence of significant differences in the incidence of angiographic CME in our study groups, we favor the maintenance of an intact capsule after extracapsular surgery, primarily because of prospective studies demonstrating a reduced incidence of retinal detachment in eyes in which the posterior capsule remains intact.

What is the incidence of clinical CME after YAG posterior capsulotomy? Various studies have reported clinical CME rates of 0.6% to 2.3% following YAG posterior capsulotomy.[32,33,34] These studies may not reflect the true incidence of clinical CME occurring in eyes which have had extracapsular surgery and posterior chamber lens implantation with intact posterior capsules and have subsequently developed capsular opacification. These are retrospective studies in which the lens type is not mentioned and/or aphakic and pseudophakic eyes are combined for reporting purposes. In fact, the true incidence of clinic CME following YAG capsulotomy may be even lower. Koch, et al.[22] retrospectively analyzed 121 eyes followed for at least one year. Although four eyes developed retinal detachments and one developed an acute symptomatic retinal tear, there were no cases of clinical CME (visual acuity 20/30 or worse). A prospective study of CME after YAG laser posterior capsulotomy was performed by Lewis et al.[35] One hundred and thirty-eight eyes of 136 consecutive patients undergoing YAG capsulotomy following cataract surgery (range, 4–54 months) had pre-laser fluorescein angiograms. Patients were examined at 24 hours, 1 week, 1 month, 3 months, and 6 months after capsulotomy. Fluorescein angiography was performed between 4 and 8 weeks after the posterior capsulotomy. Eighty eyes of 78 patients (57%) had a minimum follow-up of 6 months and underwent repeated fluorescein angiography. None of the 80 eyes showed evidence of clinical or angiographic CME. Although this study is flawed by a relatively small number of patients, it is important because it is a prospective study and patients with angiographic CME prior to capsulotomy were eliminated. One may assume that the incidence of CME following YAG laser posterior capsulotomy is quite small. If the incidence of clinical CME is truly as low as has been reported in these studies, why are implant surgeons concerned? Jampol[36] has correctly pointed out three reasons: 1) patients have been "promised" an excellent visual acuity following cataract surgery; 2) with over one million cataract procedures being performed annually, a 1% incidence of visually significant CME will result in 10,000 unhappy patients and; 3) the incidence of clinically significant CME is much greater in eyes which have had surgical complications.

In summary, retinal detachment develops in approximately 0.005 to 0.010% of phakic eyes annually. The incidence of detachment following cataract surgery is approximately 1 to 3%. This increase is primarily due to biochemical changes in the vitreous gel with a subsequent increase in the posterior vitreous detachment rate. Factors which increase the incidence of retinal detachment are axial myopia, previous history of retinal detachment, relative youth, male sex, vitreous loss and intraoperative or postoperative capsulotomy. The retinal detachment rate in myopic eyes with an intact posterior capsule is approximately 5–7%. Vitreous loss at the time of surgery increases the rate of retinal detachment significantly with various studies reporting rates of 7 to 15%. The incidence of detachment in eyes undergoing primary or a secondary capsulotomy is approximately 3%. The addition of risk factors such as myopia increase the rate to 8–10%. With additional risk factors such as relative youth and male sex associated with myopia, the rate increases to approximately 17%.

The incidence of clinical cystoid macular edema varies from less than 2% in uncomplicated cases to 18–20% in complicated cases. A primary capsulotomy has a minimal effect on the incidence of cystoid macular edema and the performance of a secondary YAG laser capsulotomy does not seem to alter the incidence figures. However, because the retinal detachment rate is increased following primary or secondary capsulotomy, it is recommended that the capsule be left intact.

References

1. Stark WJ, Sommer A, Smith RE. Changing trends in intraocular lens implantation. Editorial. Arch Ophthal 1989; 107:1441–1444.
2. Norton EW. Detachment problems related to aphakia. *Second Cataract Surgical Congress*, Miami Beach, FL: Miami Educational Press Inc; 1971:149.
3. Goldberg MF. Clear lens extraction for axial myopia. An appraisal. Ophthalmology 1987; 94:571–582.
4. Hagler WS. Pseudophakic retinal detachment. Trans Am Ophthalmol Soc 1982; 80:45–50.
5. McDonnell PJ, Patel A, and Green WR. Comparison of intracapsular and extracapsular cataract surgery. Histopathologic study of eyes obtained postmortem. Ophthalmology. 1985; 92:1208.
6. Osterlin S. Changes in the macromolecular composition of the vitreous produced by removal of the lens. In Puig Solanes M, (ed.). *Proceedings of the 21st International Congress of Ophthalmology*, Mexico, 1970. Amsterdam, Excerpta Medica, 1971:1620.
7. Osterlin S. Vitreous changes after cataract extraction. In Freeman HM, Hirose T, and Schepens CL (eds.). *Vitreous Surgery and Advances in Fundus Diagnosis and Treatment*. Boston, MA Appleton-Century-Crofts; 1975:15.
8. Kangro M, and Osterlin S. Hyaluronate concentration in the vitreous of the pseudophakic eye. *Invest Ophthal*. Vis Sci 26:(AFVO Suppl) 1985:28.
9. Michels RG, Wilkinson CP, Rice TA. *Retinal Detachment*, St. Louis, MO; Mosby Inc.: 1990.
10. Hovland KR. Vitreous findings in fellow eyes of aphakic retinal detachment. Am J Ophthalmol 1978; 86:350.
11. Ruben M, Rajpurohit P. Distribution of myopia in aphakic retinal detachments. Br J Ophthalmol 1976; 60:517–521.

12. Jaffe NS, Clayman HM, Jaffe MS. Retinal detachment in myopic eyes after intracapsular and extracapsular cataract extraction. Am J Ophthalmol 1984; 97:48–52.
13. Gross KA, Pearce JL. Modern cataract surgery in a highly myopic population. Br J Ophthalmol 1987; 71:215–219.
14. Smith PW, Stark WJ, Maumenee AE, et al. Retinal detachment after extracapsular cataract extraction with posterior chamber intraocular lens. Ophthalmology 1987; 94:495–502.
15. Lindstrom RL, Lindquist TD, Huldin J, Rubenstein JB. Retinal detachment in axial myopia following extracapsular cataract surgery. *Transactions of the New Orleans Academy of Ophthalmology*, New York: Raven Press Ltd; 1988.
16. Benson WE, Grand MG, Okun E. Aphakic retinal detachment; management of the fellow eye. Arch Ophthalmol 1975; 93:245–249.
17. Coonan P, Fung WE, Webster RG, Allen AW Jr, Abbot RL. The incidence of retinal detachment following extracapsular cataract extraction. Ophthalmology 1985; 92:1096–1101.
18. Byers NE. Changes in and prognosis of lattice degeneration of the retina. Trans Am Acad Ophthalmol Otolaryngol 1974; 78:114.
19. Wilkinson CP, Anderson LS, Little JH. Retinal detachment following phacoemulsification. Ophthalmology 85:151–56, 1978.
20. Hurite FG, Forr EM, Everett WG. The incidence of retinal detachment following phacoemulsification. Ophthalmology 1979; 86:2004–2006.
21. Troutman RC, Clahane AC, Emery JM, et al. Cataract surgery of the cataract-phacoemulsification committee. Trans Am Ophthal Otolaryngol 1975; 79:178–85.
22. Koch DD, Liu JF, Gill EP, Parke DW II. Axial myopia increases the risk of retinal complications after Neodymium-YAG laser posterior capsulotomy. Arch Ophthalmol 1989; 107:986–990.
23. Leff SR, Welch JC, Tasman W. Rhegmatogenous retinal detachment after YAG laser posterior capsulotomy. Ophthalmol 1987; 94:1222–1224.
24. Rickman-Barger L, Florine CW, Larson RS, Lindstrom RL. Retinal detachment after Neodymium-YAG laser posterior capsulotomy. Am J Ophthalmol 1989; 107:531–536.
25. Ober RR, Wilkinson CP, Fiore JV Jr, Maggiano JM. Rhegmatogenous retinal detachment after Neodymium-YAG laser capsulotomy. Phakic (sic) and pseudophakic eyes: Am J Ophthalmol 1986; 101:81–89.
26. Bradford JD, Wilkinson CP, Bradford, Jr RH. Cystoid macular edema following extracapsular cataract extraction and posterior chamber intraocular lens implantation. Retina 1988; 8:161–164.
27. Stark WJ, Maumenee AE, Fagadau W, Patiles M, Baker, et al. Cystoid macular edema in pseudophakia. Surv Ophthalmol 1984; 28:442–451.
28. Jaffe NS, Clayman HM, Jaffe MS. Cystoid macular edema after intracapsular and extracapsular cataract extraction with and without an intraocular lens. Ophthalmology 1982; 89:25–29.

29. Kraff MC, Sanders DR, Jampol LM, et al. Effect of primary capsulotomy with extracapsular surgery on the incidence of pseudophakic cystoid macular edema. Am J Ophthalmol 1984; 98:166–170.

30. Wright PL, Wilkinson CP, Balyeat HD, Popham J, Reinke M. Angiographic cystoid macular edema after posterior chamber lens implantation. Arch Ophthalmol 1988; 106:740–744.

31. Javitt JC. When does the failure to find a difference mean that there is none? Arch Ophthalmol 1989; 107:2034–2040.

32. Winslow RL, Taylor BC. Retinal complications following YAG laser capsulotomy. Ophthalmology 1985; 92:785–789.

33. Keates RH, Steinhert RF, Puliafito CA, Maxwell SK. Long-term follow up of Nd:YAG laser posterior capsulotomy. J Am Intraocul Implant Soc 1984; 10:164–68.

34. Shah GR, Gills JP, Durham DG, Ausmus WH. Three thousand YAG lasers in posterior capsulotomies: An analysis of complications and comparison to polishing and surgical discussions. Ophthalmic Surg 1986; 17:473–477.

35. Lewis H, Singer TR, Hanscom TA, Straatsma BR. A prospective study of cystoid macular edema after Neodymium:YAG laser posterior capsulotomy. Ophthalmology 1987; 94:478–482.

36. Jampol LM. Cystoid macular edema following cataract surgery. Editorial. Arch Ophthalmol 1988; 106:894–895

ROUNDTABLE DISCUSSION MANAGEMENT OF CATARACT PATIENTS WITH SMALL PUPILS AND/OR GLAUCOMA

Hal D. Balyeat, MD, Moderator

Balyeat: What I would like to do is talk about some cases involving small pupils in individuals with glaucoma. I think this is a very pertinent topic. We face these patients daily in our practice and, invariably, we have some problems that arise. What I'll do is present some case histories, or patient presentations, and we can get the panel members to discuss their feelings about this.

First, we have a 74-year-old white female with a 20-year history of chronic open-angle glaucoma. She has been controlled all these years on pilocarpine four times a day. She has a relatively dense nuclear sclerotic cataract and a minimal amount of cupping. Assuming that this patient has a relatively small pupil from her many years of miotics, Cal, I might ask you how you would proceed with her.

Roberts: This time we are talking in terms of the pupil, and not in terms of the corneal endothelium. What I try to do is, since I don't like a lot of surprises in the O.R., I'll try to make a really valiant attempt at dilating her pre-operatively to just get a feeling of what I can expect in the O.R. Basically, in the O.R. I do one of two things. I either try to stretch the pupil in cases where the pupil is smaller than I feel adequate, or the other situation which I do is to make a radial incision at 12 o'clock and preplace a 10-0 prolene to keep the pupil, therefore, open throughout the case. At the end, I sew it closed. That's a technique that I've been doing for a while and it works well. But I use it only in cases where I can't stretch the pupil.

Balyeat: Bill?

Simcoe: Well, I do it very similarly. I share Cal's dislike for surprises in the operating room. If they'll dilate up enough and I think I can get them out, then I'll try. Some years ago I would spend lots of time trying to deliver one through a relatively small pupil like a breech birth, I suppose, and as Henry Hirschman referred to his invincible period, I was able to get some of them out through some pretty small pupils. I've found that I stretched the pupils sometimes permanently. The pupil became somewhat flaccid and sort of non-responsive when it would come back down later because I had actually fractured it. It was also more prone to synechiae and didn't look as good. So, do what Cal suggested which is to make a little peripheral iridectomy and then slide a scissors through it and make a radial cut. Actually, I will sew the iris at the end of the procedure. I like to bring the pupils back down to normal size and relatively normal shape—not only cosmetically, but functionally—because people don't like the glare and image problems of a sector iridectomy. So, what you can do is gently go into the eye, and particularly if you have Healon, (or under an air bubble), pull one pillar of iris just to the lip of the wound and pass your suture from beneath it forward. Then, push the iris back in; pull the other pillar out; pass your suture from forward, backwards, then tie up your repaired iris ends.

Balyeat: I would echo those sentiments. I think that this is particularly important for the residents. The residents are always concerned about how those eyes look when their peers examine them, and they want to be sure that those pupils are nice and round. They sometimes find themselves in significant problems because one, the pupil is miotic. They try to do a small capsulotomy and end up with significant large capsular flaps that they have to deal with. Then they stretch the pupil and they end up with a flaccid iris, particularly in an elderly blue-eyed patient. They have all these capsular tags that they're dealing with when they're doing their aspiration and cortical clean-up, and they end up tearing the capsule. I think that it behooves them and all of us when there is any question at all about the pupillary size, that it is prudent to simply do a sphincterotomy and then either close it or leave it open. I would agree that most of the time we'll close those, but there are occasional patients who may be highly myopic or they have other retinal problems in the past, and we can leave those open and usually not have too much trouble with glare.

Simcoe: Incidentally, Hal, later if the retina surgeon needs to have a better view, you can pop that suture later with a laser.

Balyeat: Right. This next patient is a 65-year-old lady with a history of chronic open-angle glaucoma. This woman is poorly controlled on medication—pilocarpine and beta-blockers. She's intolerant to carbonic anhydrase inhibitors and has a significant cataract with some visual field loss and the pressures are higher than one would like. How would you handle this case? Cal?

Roberts: I am going to borrow a phrase of Bill's, that "This is a situation in which you need a real doctor." I have gotten burned by these cases enough that anyone like this I send to our glaucoma specialist. In the first place, without a trabeculectomy the day after surgery, these patients have pressures that are 38mmHg or 40mmHg. On the other hand, some of the patients with trabeculectomies develop flat chambers. This is not where I'm at my best and so I send them absolutely to a glaucoma person, let them make the decision and let them be there to do what has to be done.

Balyeat: Would their decision, in your experience, usually be to do a combined procedure?

Roberts: Yes, they usually do.

Simcoe: I don't do combined procedures, and probably it's how you're taught. I trained at the University of Pennsylvania and it was felt, at that time 30 years ago when I was there, that glaucoma should always be controlled before cataract surgery. Well, of course, that was intracapsular days and we didn't have a lot of the things that we now have, but I've always been sort of afraid to combine surgery. I've done it two or three times and gotten by, but I have seen cases that got into real trouble—luckily not my own cases, so, what I would do is probably a bit old fashioned. I would go ahead and do the filtration surgery if that's what it took. I let that eye quiet down and maintain the bleb well. Six or eight weeks later, I would then do extracapsular extraction with a lens implant following surgical control of the glaucoma.

I would like to mention briefly something that I learned years ago that has been a life saver for me. I was taught a long time ago that when blebs would close off, do digital pressure. Well, I found that the patients wouldn't do it because it hurt them. This is because you are pushing up where the incision is. I have seen cases where you could prolapse vitreous and have all kinds of problems in doing that. So, many years ago, I began using my own technique routinely on all of my post-filtering glaucoma patients after a few days when their pressure began to get up in the normal range or in the teens. I have them close their eye and apply the hypothenar eminence of their hand gently to push back until they just almost feel discomfort. It is a diffuse pressure; it doesn't hurt the eye, and I have them do that five or 10 seconds on and off. We'd teach them in the office and monitor their pressure like a hawk. I had a woman in her twenties come in who had had multiple surgical procedures for juvenile glaucoma. She had had goniotomy and several filtering operations with both eye pressures up near 40mmHg. She was going blind. I filtered both eyes—the last one five years ago. With gentle massage, twice a day, her pressures remain in the low teens. It's a nice trick.

Balyeat: I'm glad to see that Bill and I are consistent, because I do a lot of combined procedures! I think that they are useful. I think that there is an increased morbidity with these patients, so you have to exercise a lot of care and you have to be ready to have some increased hyphemas. I think a real nice trick is to do a phacoemulsification on these patients.

You can usually do this superotemporally. Do a trabeculectomy at the same time; go through the trabeculectomy site with the ultrasound tip. Oftentimes you have to do a sphincterotomy. You can then have a trabeculectomy in a quadrant so if the trabeculectomy does fail you can go ahead and do a second trabeculectomy if necessary, usually in the superonasal quadrant. So, it is one of the advantages. Although I do a fair amount of planned extracapsular surgery as well as phacoemulsification, I think that this is one situation where phacoemulsification is a useful tool.

Roberts: If you're going through your trabeculectomy site, don't you have an increased iris prolapse?

Balyeat: Not if I've done a sphincterotomy. In other words, you can blow the iris away with the viscoelastic and it really keeps it out of the way pretty well.

Simcoe: I have no quarrel with combined procedures. Many people do them and they work well, it's just kind of how I was raised.

Balyeat: Let's go on. Here's a lady with a cataract who has had a previous filter which is working reasonably well. She has to use some medication for control, but she has a nice filter that is visualized easily superiorly, and her pupil dilates well. Cal?

Roberts: I would want to do specular microscopy and make sure that she has a reasonable endothelial reserve. With a patient like this I would make a clear corneal incision and try to stay away from her trabeculectomy site.

Balyeat: Bill?

Simcoe: I, too, would do her cataract operation. I would start over with my incision at the normal place—the posterior surgical limbus—then as I approach the bleb I would go in front of it. I wouldn't make an entirely corneal incision, but basically do the same thing Cal's doing.

Balyeat: I think it is of interest—I know there are a lot of people who go through filtering blebs to do their procedure. That never has made a lot of sense to me, and I too go in clear cornea in front of the bleb. I think there is an occasional time when you have some of these blebs that may have been done with unguarded procedures and are very succulent, and you may have to go through the bleb in a situation like that. But that is a very rare situation. I generally use interrupted 10-0 nylon in these situations, as opposed to prolene or mersilene for two reasons: one is that the knots are softer and you can bury them, and secondly, if you do have some induced astigmatism and you have to take out sutures, it's nice to have the interrupted sutures as opposed to a running suture.

Roberts: Also, the knots of the sutures are going to tend to tear at the cornea, and if you use a prolene or mersilene suture you'll actually see a tear. The nylon will stretch.

Balyeat: Here we have an 80 year old individual with a previous filter, only this individual is poorly controlled on maximum medication with significant cupping and visual field constriction. This is a variation of the patient that was just presented. Bill, how would you attack that?

Simcoe: I would send her to you!

Balyeat: Thanks a lot for your confidence! Cal?

Roberts: I think a patient like this definitely needs to get filtered before-hand, and make sure the pressure is under control before doing your cataract surgery. Certainly, the cataract surgery is elective and if you are not able to control her intraocular pressure, and you are seeing disc changes and visual field changes, that is certainly the higher priority than is her cataract.

Balyeat: So, you would suggest either doing or having some sort of fil-tration surgery done and not combined; then go back in and do a clear corneal section at a later date?

Roberts: That's right.

Simcoe: Well, I was being a little facetious a while ago, but not entirely. I would like to address the young surgeons with something about responsibility. Sure, I could go in and I might do another filter on this one, because since it's uncontrolled, by my own simple definition it means that filter isn't working and it isn't going to work adequately. So, I would agree with Cal to do it again. Since we have an institute at home that is a very good one with good facilities, I would face a moral decision. I have to decide if I am going to go in and operate on this patient again, and then if I fail, what do I do? I then decide to send the patient to the institute and let them wrestle with another failed attempt—or should I, at that point, decide to let them make the initial decision and not have another go at the surgery? Now, I'm talking to the young surgeons. Somewhere along the line, you have to start looking down the road where if you really are going to have a possible nightmare on your hands, when do you ask for help? It might be a courtesy to first get the consultation from the people into whose lap you might dump the problem, and let them be involved in the decision making, rather than get into trouble and say, "Here you are."

Balyeat: Good point. This is an individual that we saw recently who was fairly perplexing. This patient had a significant amount of angle recession following trauma years ago. The patient also had a markedly elevated intraocular pressure on maximum medications; had a significant cataract, and also had a partial dislocation of the zonules inferiorly. Do any of you have any suggestions? Go ahead, Cal.

Roberts: I think my feelings are similar to the patient before. Again, the highest priority is getting the pressure down so that this would not be a patient that I would be taking care of. It would be somebody that a glaucoma person would be handling.

Simcoe: We haven't mentioned whether any laser was tried. I assume on all of these that they've tried maximum medication?

Balyeat: Yes.

Simcoe: This patient will have to be filtered. Obviously, this one is going to be a tough one. This is one that you are going to be really worried about. You are going to be worried about any external pressure afterwards, too, like I do. This type of patient should see the specialist.

Balyeat: One of the problems that we are confronted with in these kinds of patients is what happens if you have vitreous loss, and this is a typical example of what might happen. I think this patient is a prime candidate no matter how well the cataract procedure is done. So then, you've got vitreous in the anterior chamber; perhaps you have a functioning bleb prior to that time. I would make a point. I think that a vitrectomy done correctly is not a reason for a filter to fail. It is a fact that during a combined cataract operation and filter, or in light of a previous filter, oftentimes the vitrectomy is inadequately performed and then vitreous gets into the anterior chamber. So, I would make a plea in a situation like this for a pars plana vitrectomy. I think you certainly may not want to do it yourself, but this may be a situation in which you can remove all the vitreous and not jeopardize the filter.

Simcoe: The moral there is like many things in life. Once you make the decision to do something, then do it adequately. Don't go in and meddle about a bit and stir up the vitreous and say, "Gee, I've helped this a lot!" Get rid of it.

Roberts: This is also a situation in which I would not do phacoemulsification. Dislocations like these I've found have been very, very difficult to do with a phaco, and I would be much more likely to do either planned extracapsular—if I thought I could do it—or go ahead and do an intracapsular.

Balyeat: It is interesting. I think that phaco surgeons, the ones who do a tremendous amount of phaco, would say that this was exactly the kind of patient that ought to be done with phacoemulsification, and would propose that it be done that way.

This next patient is a fairly typical patient who has a peripheral iridectomy combined with a sphincterotomy and the iris closed (Figure 8-1). I do pretty much like Bill does and grab the iris pillars. After the procedure I don't like to have anything in the anterior chamber that I might get hung up on, like a suture, and it's nice to be able to blow back that iris with the viscoelastic and then have a nice, large area so you can do a good capsulotomy.

Simcoe: Those of you who have done this fairly often, realize that no matter how you try you will sometimes have a little unevenness of the pupil, like right up at the top. I do; we all do. The point I want to make is I would put in a second suture, usually further up. It is really not that hard to do. While it may be nit-picky, I think it probably helps some of the glare and problems—you know that amount of the iridectomy visible is exposed. It's not underneath the lid. So, I put a second one right up there where it kind of makes a "Y."

Roberts: I think a little difference in my technique is I don't put my suture close to the pupil. For me it's about 1.5mm back. So there is actually a little gap right at the pupil, but it is a little more secure posteriorly.

Balyeat: I think it important to re-emphasize this. Please do perform sphincterotomies whenever there is any question at all. This slide (Figure 8-2) is the way we want all of them to look. Unfortunately,

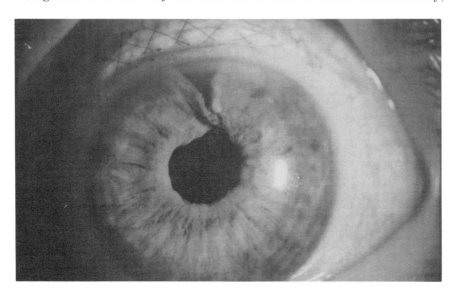

Figure 8-1:   Peripheral iridectomy combined with a sphincterotomy and sutured iris.

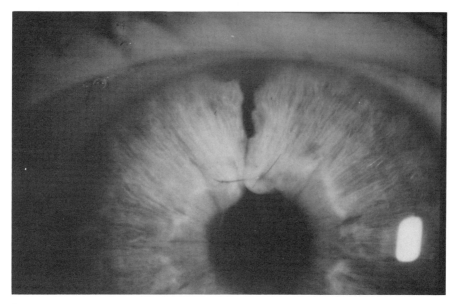

Figure 8-2: Excellent desired result following suturing of sphincterotomy.

they are not always that nice. They oftentimes can be more like this (Figure 8-3), particularly if you have a patient with a flaccid iris and some iris atrophy. I still don't think you have to be so concerned about the appearance of the pupil. What you are trying to do is get a functional result. This is a patient (Figure 8-4) in whom a cataract extraction was done by method we were talking about before. This gentle-

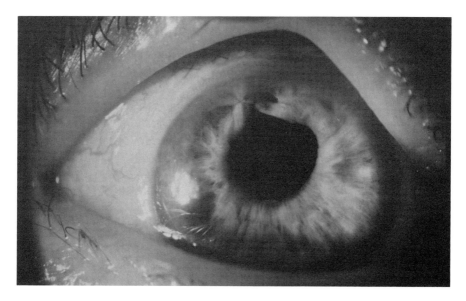

Figure 8-3: Corectopion following cataract extraction due to flaccid iris.

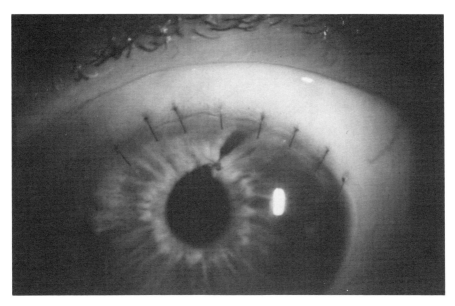

Figure 8-4:   Patient showing preferred method of leaving existing filtering bleb alone in which incision is made anterior to the filter along with sphincterotomy and iris suturing.

man—it's his only eye—has a nice filtering bleb. The incision was made through clear cornea; a sphincterotomy was performed, and then the clear corneal incision was closed with interrupted nylon as you can see there. Thank you very much.

Chapter 9

EXPERIENCE WITH MULTIFOCAL IOLs

Howard V. Gimbel, MD

Visual and Refractive Results of a Large Series of 3M Multifocal IOLS

With the advent of modern microsurgical techniques, good functional visual acuity can be obtained in the majority of IOL cases. Visual distortions from aphakic spectacle correction and the inconveniences of contact lenses have largely been overcome. However, pseudophakia is still associated with a loss of accommodative ability, and bifocal contact lenses have been less than optimal. Bifocal spectacle reading glasses have been the mainstays allowing distance and near vision in the pseudophakic patient. The loss of accommodative ability associated with standard lenses is an issue that is being addressed by the development of IOLs that create more than one focal point to approximate the accommodation power of the phakic eye.

The simplest bifocal lens design introduced recently is the IOLAB two-zone refractive IOL. (Figure 9-1) This lens has one power in the periphery for distance vision and a higher power (+ 3) in the central portion of near vision. For example, if a lens power of 20 D is recommended for emmetropia, the lens implanted would have a power of 20 D in the periphery and 23 D in the center. (Figure 9-2) One of the possible disadvantages of this design is that if the pupil dilates, for instance in low light, more light will enter the distance portion, overwhelming the near image.

Pharmacia has developed a lens that is very similar to the IOLAB design, but it has a distance portion in the center of the lens, with the near portion around that, and another distance portion in the periphery. This "donut-hole" design should allow for adequate light to the distance focus when the pupil aperture is very small. However, the problem of adequate light to the near focus when the pupil is dilated remains. Also, how decentration would affect vision is not known.

Dr. Lee Nordan has developed an aspheric lens design which creates an infinite number of focal points. Figure 9-3 shows the difference between an aspheric curve and a spherical curve. Each location on the aspheric curve has a slightly different curvature, and therefore, a different refrac-

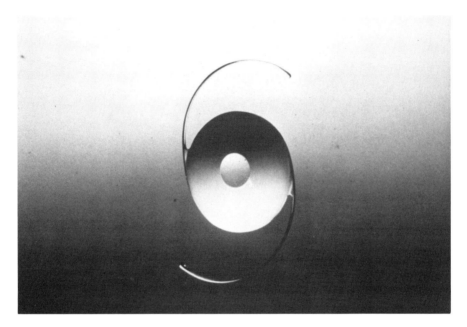

Figure 9-1: IOLAB bifocal 2-zone refractive IOL

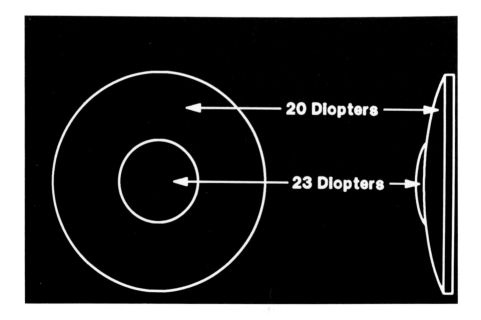

Figure 9-2: Bifocal lens design

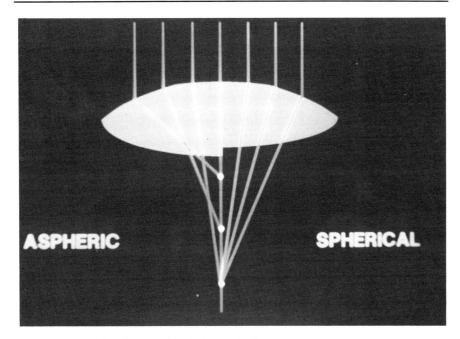

Figure 9-3:   Nordan aspheric lens design

tive power. There are two styles of Nordan multifocal lenses. Style I, (Figure 9-4) manufactured by Wright Medical is a silicone Sinskey-style PC IOL. It has a semicircular aspheric portion dedicated to near vision. Style II, (Figure 9-5) manufactured by IOPTEX, is a PMMA PC IOL with the spherical and aspheric curves combined so that no transition lines are present. The aspheric portion is placed in a donut-hole configuration. Data on the Nordan lenses remains limited.

Recently, 3M/Vision Care reported promising results with a new multifocal IOL design based on both refractive and diffractive optics. (Figure 9–6) Refraction is the bending of light rays at a smooth, continuous optical surface. (Figure 9–7) A conventional IOL uses refractive optics to bend the light to a single focal point. When discontinuities exist on the surface on the order of magnitude of a wavelength of light, the light acts like a wave rather than just a ray. Then, diffractive optics come into play. (Figure 9–8) The light wave can be out of phase, causing destructive interference (Figure 9–9), or in phase, causing constructive interference (Figure 9–10). The focal points are those regions where the light waves are in phase.

The 3M multifocal IOL (Figures 9–11 and 9–12) uses 20 to 30 concentric zones to form a diffractive structure. The lens creates two orders of diffraction, 0 and 1, and thus two focal points. The zero order of diffraction allows light to enter unimpeded by the diffraction so the normal refractive power of the lens determines the focal point. The first order of diffraction couples the refractive power with the diffraction to create a second focal point. Forty-one percent of the light is focused at the first focal point, 41% at the second, and 18% of the light is scattered.

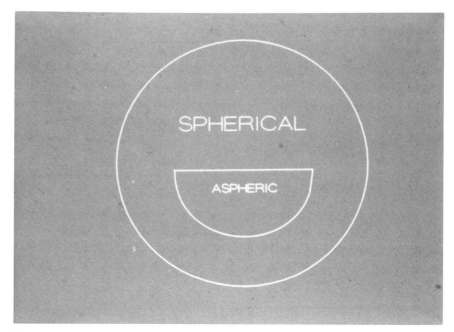

Figure 9-4: Nordan Style I

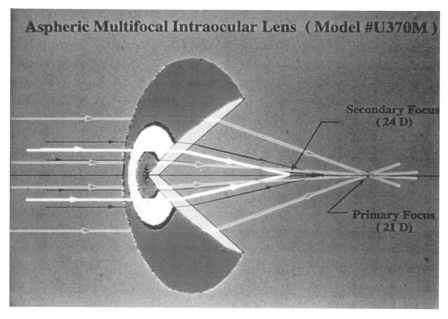

Figure 9-5: Nordan Style II

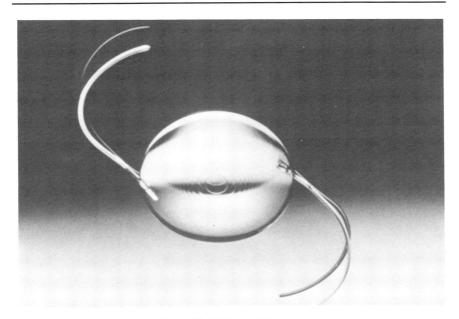

Figure 9-6:   3M/Vision Care Multifocal IOL

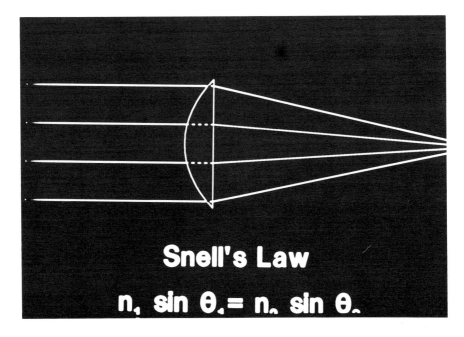

Figure 9-7:   Refraction-bending of light rays

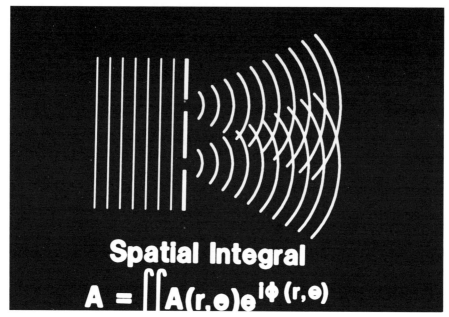

Figure 9-8:   Diffraction

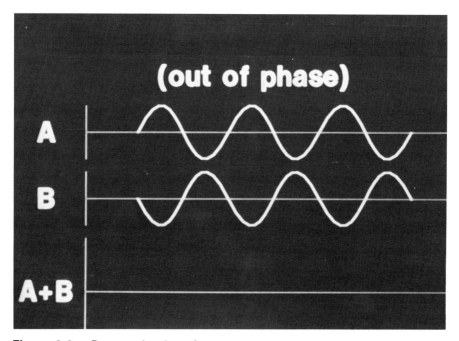

Figure 9-9:   Destructive interference

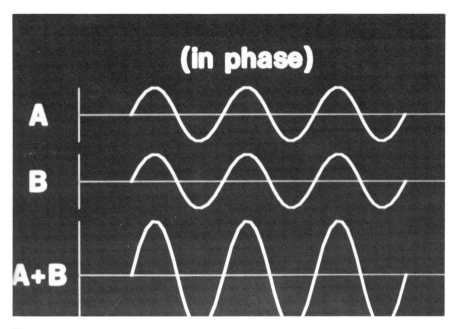

Figure 9-10:   Constructive interference

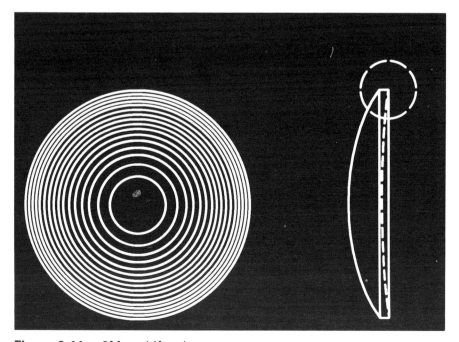

Figure 9-11:   3M multifocal

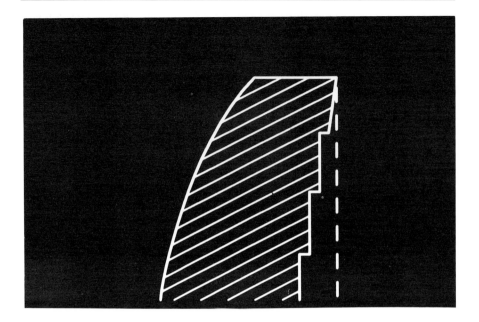

Figure 9-12:   Zone step detail—3M multifocal

For example, suppose the lens had a base power of 20 diopters, with an added power of 3 diopters for near vision. For distance vision, the share of light at the 20 D focal point is focused at the retina, so that is the image that is perceived. For near vision, the light at the 23 D focal point is focused at the retina. The image at the other focal point is too defocused to be perceived. Theoretically, one of the possible disadvantages of multifocal IOLs is the loss of contrast sensitivity in low light, as the available light is split between the two focal points (Figure 9–13).

One possible advantage of the 3M design is that every portion of the lens is used for both focal points, so the amount of light for each focus is independent of pupil dilation. Figure 9–14 shows that a pupil size changes from bright light to low light, the percent of light at the distance or near focus changes in the IOLAB and Pharmacia designs, whereas the percent of light at the two focci is evenly split at any pupil size in the 3M design.

We have been implanting 3M bifocal lenses since March 1989. By December 7, 1989 we had implanted 434 lenses including 108 bilateral cases. As of that cutoff date, we had 8–week follow-up on 140 cases and 3–month follow-up on 52 cases. Of 140 cases with at least 8–week follow-up, 113 had uncorrected distance vision of 20/40 or better (Figure 9–15). Thirty-four were seeing 20/20 or better. One hundred thirty-seven had best corrected vision of 20/40 or better (Figure 9–16), and 95 had corrected vision of 20/20 or better. Patients with small degrees of astigmatism or macular degeneration were not excluded.

Using the Jaeger acuity chart, 97 patients saw the J4 line or better with no correction in place, and 61 saw the J2 line or better. (Figure 9–17) With distance correction in place, 100 could see the J4 line or better

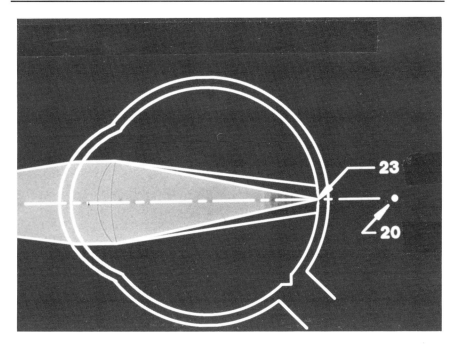

Figure 9-13:   Loss of contrast sensitivity in multifocal IOL due to splitting of light between two focal points.

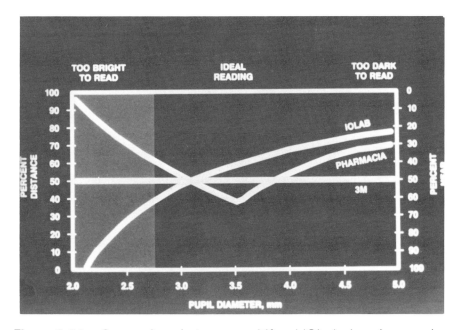

Figure 9-14:   Comparison between multifocal IOL designs in regard to pupil size and perceived brightness.

>-20/20	34 (24.3%)
>-20/25	68 (48.6%)
>-20/30	94 (67.1%)
>-20/40	113 (80.7%)

Figure 9-15: Distance vision uncorrected > 8 weeks postop

>-20/20	99 (70.7%)
>-20/25	115 (82.1%)
>-20/30	129 (92.1%)
>-20/40	137 (97.8%)

Figure 9-16: Distance vision best corrected > 8 weeks postop

>-J2	61 (43.6%)
>-J3	79 (56.4%)
>-J4	97 (69.3%)

Figure 9-17: Near vision uncorrected > 8 weeks postop

and 78 could see the J2 or better (Figure 9–18). Mean spherical equivalent was -0.36 D, ranging from -2.63 D to 2.26 D (Figure 9–19). The mean preoperative keratometric cylinder was 0.63 D, ranging from 0 D to 2.13 D. The mean postoperative keratometric cylinder was 0.98 D, ranging from 0 D to 2.87 D. (Figure 9–20) The mean change in cylinder was 0.47 D, ranging from 0 D to 1.63 D. (Figure 9–21)

As we mentioned earlier, we have 108 bilateral multifocal cases. Of these 108 cases, 80 were eligible for a subjective patient assessment questionnaire designed by 3M. Patients with any preop pathologies, including macular degeneration were eliminated. Of the 80 eligible patients, we were successful in reaching 59 by phone; 57 had usable data.

Examining 5–6 week postoperative results for these bilateral cases, mean spherical equivalence was +0.10 D, ranging from -1.00 to +1.125 D, (Figure 9–22) with a mean absolute deviation of 0.39 D and a standard deviation of 0.49 D. (Figure 9–23) A control monofocal group had a mean spherical equivalence of -0.55 D, ranging from -3.375 D to +1.125 D and a standard deviation of 0.69 D. The mean postop cylinder in the multifocal group was -0.67 D, ranging from 0.0 D to -2.00 D, with a standard devia-

>-J2	78 (55.7%)
>-J3	88 (62.8%)
>-J4	100 (71.4%)

Figure 9-18: Near vision with distance correction > 8 weeks postop

MEAN	− 0.36 D
MAX	+ 2.26 D
MIN	− 2.63 D

Figure 9-19: Spherical equivalent

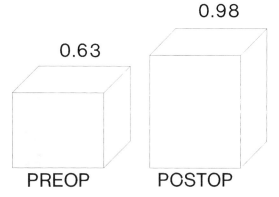

0.98

0.63

PREOP   POSTOP

Figure 9-20: Mean Keratometric cylinder

MEAN CHANGE	0.47 D
MAX CHANGE	1.63 D
MIN CHANGE	0 D

Figure 9-21: Mean change in cylinder

MEAN SPHERICAL EQUIVALENT	+ 0.10 D
MAX	+ 1.125 D
MIN	− 1.00 D

Figure 9-22: Mean spherical equivalent

MAD	—	0.39
SD	—	0.49
SEE	—	0.06

Figure 9-23:   Bilateral deviation

tion of 0.57 D. The mean postop cylinder in the control monofocal group was -0.90 D, ranging from 0.0 D to -2.50 D, with a standard deviation of 0.64 D.

We chose a concurrent, age and sex matched series of monofocal controls, who were also contracted to answer the patient satisfaction questionnaire. (Figures 9-24 and 9-25) Patients were asked if they could see near and distance objects clearly, in daylight, with their glasses on. Almost every respondent could see distant objects clearly (96–98%). However, more multifocal cases could see near objects clearly, compared with monofocal cases (Figure 9-26) and there were no reported differences between monofocal and multifocal cases with respect to the quality of near or distance vision in either low or bright light.

Both groups rated their overall vision similarly, with 95–97% rating their vision as good to excellent. (Figure 9-27) 12.5% of multifocal patients reported blurred distance vision compared to 0% of the monofocal cases. (Figure 9-28) In addition, close to half of all multifocal cases reported seeing rings and halos, compared with only 9% of monofocal cases. These differences were statistically significant. Significantly more multifocal cases reported problems with night vision both in general and for those who drove, with night driving. (Figure 9-29 and 9-30) There were no

MULTI CASES	57
MONO CONTROLS	57
	114

Figure 9-24:   Bilateral case patient satisfaction survey

	%M	%F	MEAN AGE
MULTI	39%	61%	73
MONO	37%	63%	74

Figure 9-25:   Age/sex matched

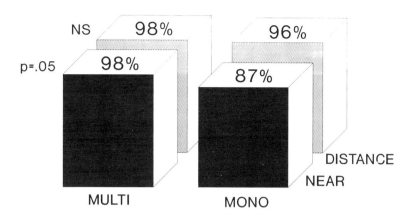

Figure 9-26:   Percentage of cases with clear vision

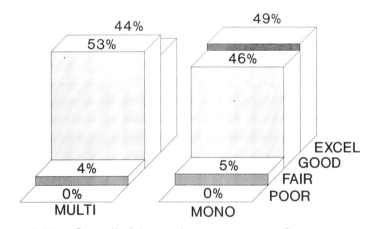

Figure 9-27:   Overall vision rating-percentage of cases

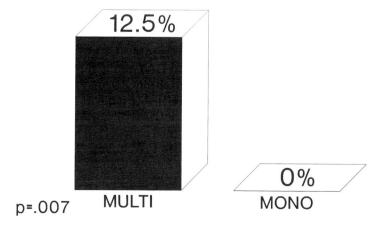

Figure 9-28:   Blurred distance vision-percentage of cases

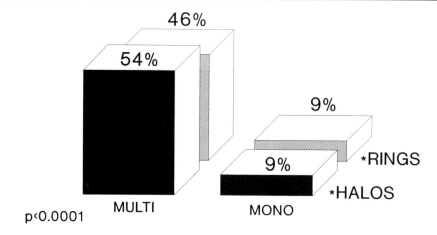

Figure 9-29:   Rings and/or halos-percentage of cases

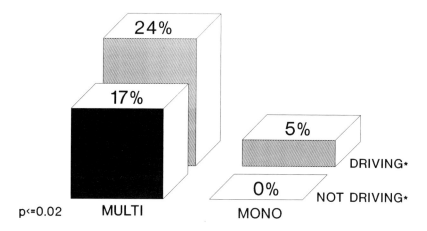

Figure 9-30:   Problems with night vision-percentage of cases

group differences in the proportion of cases reporting flare, glare, near vision distortion or blurring, or diplopia. (Figure 9-31)

We believe that the halos seen at night are not strictly related to the diffractive optics of the lens design. The halo effect results when distance light passing through the near focal point reaches the retina out-of-focus and is spread diffusely around the fovea. The diffractive plates of the 3M multifocal lens spread the light from point source light into rather discrete rings of light. We have implanted a small number of IOLAB bifocal lenses and find that these patients also see a halo, but in the form of a circular glow rather than discrete rings of light. This is attributable to the IOLAB bifocal lens design spreading the light in a uniform pattern around the fovea, rather than in concentric rings.

The reason why this effect is noticeable, for example from oncoming car headlights when driving at night on a highway in complete darkness more so than on a city street, is because the retina is not illuminated

REPORTING	MULTI	MONO
FLARE/GLARE	28%	21%
NEAR VISION DISTORTION	11%	4%
NEAR VISION BLUR	14%	9%
DIPLOPIA	13%	7%
NO SIGNIFICANT DIFFERENCES		

Figure 9-31:   Additional aesthopia—percentage of cases reported.

except at the fovea and the area surrounding it. The faintness of the halo or rings seen is because of out-of-focus light being spread over a relatively large parafoveal area being compared to the concentration of the focused light on the fovea.

The appearance of halos around light at night will vary somewhat depending on the optics of the multifocal lens, but because it is related to the multiple foci of the lens it can be expected with any multifocal intraocular lens.

The distributions of spectacle status, as expected, were different between the groups. 70% of multifocal and only 9% of monofocal cases needed no spectacle correction at all. 73% of monofocal cases needed bi- or trifocals compared with 18% of multifocal cases. Likewise, the two groups were easily differentiated by their ability to function comfortably without glasses for near, intermediate, and distance vision: 91% of multifocal cases and only 35% of monofocal cases functioned well for near vision. Multifocal cases responded similarly for all distances; monofocal cases functioned better with intermediate or distance vision than for near vision. (Figure 9-32) 94% of monofocal cases and 23% of multifocal cases reported wearing bifocal or reading glasses or using a magnifier while reading. (Figure 9-33).

Our evaluation of the 3M diffractive lens is still preliminary at this point. Other investigators have reported on prospective studies comparing the 3M lens with monofocal lenses. Dr. Akel El-Maghraby has reported on a randomized study with 70 patients enrolled. At 2–4 months post-op, near vision, both uncorrected and with distance correction in place, was better for 3M cases. None of the monofocal cases could see the J1 line uncorrected, while 25% of the 3M cases could. (Figures 9-34 and 9-35)

In a multicenter trial with 16 investigators and 301 3M lenses implanted, 70.3% of patients achieved functional near acuity without additional add at 2–4 months postop, as reported by Dr. John Hunkeler. Contrast sensitivity testing showed no functional difference between multifocal and monofocal cases, and in glare testing, multifocal cases consistently scored better. (Figure 9–36) In a study by Dr.S. Piers Percival of 55 3M cases

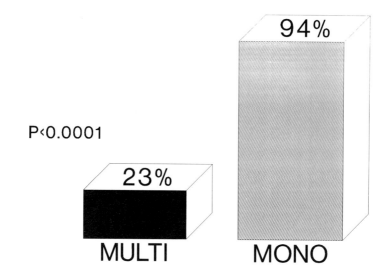

Figure 9-32:   Percentage of cases able to function comfortably without spectacles.

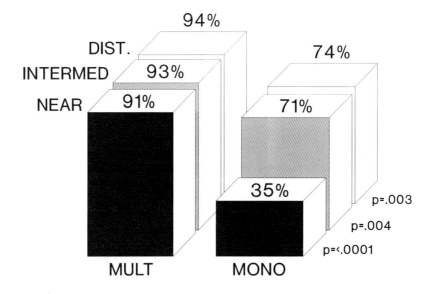

Figure 9-33:   Percentage of cases requiring reading correction.

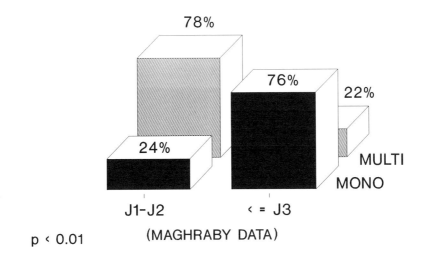

Figure 9-34:   Near acuity with distance correction.

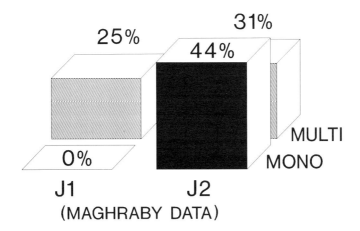

Figure 9-35:   Percentage of cases with near vision J1 and J2

- 70.3% FUNCTIONAL NEAR ACUITY
- NO DIFFERENCE IN CONTRAST SENSITIVITY
- GLARE SCORES BETTER FOR MULTIFOCAL EYES

  (MULTICENTER TRIAL REPORTED BY JOHN HUNKELER, MD)

Figure 9-36:   Results of multicenter trial of 301 3M lenses.

- BETTER NEAR ACUITY FOR
  MULTIFOCAL EYES

- PATIENT ASSESSMENT MIXED

- POOR VISION IN LOW LIGHT

- BLURRING OF NEAR VISION

  (S. PIERS PERCIVAL, MD)

Figure 9-37:   Results of 55 3M cases versus 55 monofocal cases

matched with 55 monofocal cases, 81% of the bifocal eyes could see J5 or better, while only 21% of monofocal eyes could. However, only 75% of multifocal patients rated their satisfaction as good, citing poor reading vision in dim light and blurring of near vision. (Figure 9–37)

Our patients have achieved good functional results with the 3M diffractive lens in both distance and near vision. Our results in this regard agree well with other reports in the literature on this lens.

Chapter 10

SURFACE MODIFICATIONS
OF IOLs

John D. Hunkeler, MD

In the quest for the "ideal" intraocular lens, investigators are experimenting with various modifications to the time proven polymethylmethacrylate (PMMA) surface of IOLs in an attempt to decrease or eliminate intraocular trauma and inflammation.

Herbert Kaufman first showed the deleterious effects that contact between the hydrophobic PMMA implant and the hydrophilic cornea could have on endothelial cell counts, as measured by specular microscopy. Following this study, the discovery and use of viscoelastic substances have reduced cell loss from contact of PMMA with the endothelium. Initial in vitro studies showed a reduction of cell loss from 40% to 7%. This is because viscoelastics convert the hydrophobic surface of PMMA, which is known to cause endothelial cell membrane stripping, to a hydrophilic surface which is less traumatic to endothelial cell touch. Since these discoveries, there have been a number of surface modification techniques developed to improve the biocompatibility of PMMA. Two of these techniques include heparin grafting and surface passivation of intraocular lenses.

Surface modification of PMMA using heparin causes the lens material to become hydrophilic, which results in less damage to the endothelial cells during corneal contact as well as less granulocyte activation, reduced granulocyte adhesion, and fewer deposits of foreign body giant cells.

Rabbit studies have shown a significant reduction of cell growth on the central portion of heparin-modified IOLs after three weeks of implantation. Similar results were seen in monkey studies showing less trauma to endothelial cells one year postoperatively. Clinical studies done by Fagerholm et al. and Steinkogler et al. showed a reduction in postoperative inflammation, reduction in posterior synechiae formation, and reduction in cell/pigment deposition. An explanation of these reductions may be that activation of C3 complement is less likely with heparin-modified IOLs than with PMMA alone. These studies suggest an improvement in biocompatibility through the hydrophilization of the PMMA surface with heparin.

Surface passivation, on the other hand, involves a sequence of proprietary processes involving a fluorocarbon reagent that rearranges the cellular structure on the surface of the implant. This surface passivation of the lathe-cut PMMA IOL reduces the surface energy of the implant and reduces the biological interaction of cell adherance. The series of chemical processes involved does not add any new surface material. Passivation probably involves a reduction in the number of surface defect sites, preventing protein, fats, or other cellular material to adhere to the IOL surface. This was reflected in clinical trials that showed drastically reduced adherance of endothelial cells during corneal touch. In surface passivation the actual molecules of the implant are restructured to form a smooth surface compared to the irregular untouched PMMA surface. Preliminary testing using the atomic force microscope (AFM) by Vincent McKory, Ph.D. indicates that surface passivated IOL topography is approximately twice as smooth as a nonsurface passivated lens implant. Surface energy studies show that surface modification renders the lens surface oleophobic or lipophobic. Blood and plasma adhesion studies show that significantly fewer cells and proteins adhere to the surface of modified vs. control IOLs. Additional studies seem to support the belief that these modified lenses cause less iris chafing and loss of iris pigment epithelium. Moreover, since the passivated haptic surface remains largely free of tissue interaction, biodegradation and biooxidation should be reduced.

Ioptex sponsored a large, double-blind, multicentered clinical study using a 7 mm PMMA three-piece IOL with surface passivation and prolene haptics. One hundred forty six patients were monitored over a one year period checking such parameters as visual acuity, glare disability, specular microscopy, fluorescein angiography, and complications. The results of this study showed that visual acuity was no different at eight weeks, six months, or one year postoperatively compared to normal PMMA lenses. Glare disability index testing showed a slight advantage of the passivated lenses. The incidence of endothelial cell loss, corneal edema, and posterior capsular opacification were slightly less for the passivated lenses.

Overall, there are some potential benefits in surface modifications of PMMA IOLs. These include slightly reduced endothelial cell loss, reduced pigment dispersion and iritis in the initial postoperative period, reduced instance of secondary glaucoma, reduced cystoid macular edema, and reduced glare disability. However, there still remains the question whether the expense of such modifications warrant their slight advantages. This fact is especially important in light of the declining reimbursement system. Future investigation holds the answer whether such lenses are indicated in all cataract patients or whether they should be limited to those patients in high risk groups.

References

1. Kaufman, HE, Katz J, Valenti J, Sheets JW, Goldberg EB. Corneal endothelium damage with intraocular lenses: contact adhesion between surgical materials and tissue, Science. 1977; 198:525.

2. Thunberg L, Backstrom G, Lindahl U. Further characterization of the anti-thrombin-blinding sequence in heparin. Carbohydr Res. 1982; 100:393.

3. Olsson P, Larm O, Larsson P, Lind LE, Nilsson E, Swedenborg J. Requirements for thromboresistance for surface-heparinized materials. Ann NY Acad Sci. 1983; 416:525.

4. Larsson R, Ericsson JC, Lagergren H, Olsson P. Platelet and plasma coagulation compatibility of heparinized and sulphated surfaces. Thromb Res. 1979; 15:157.

5. Fagerholm P, Lydahl E, Philipson B. Heparin surface modified lenses-an update. Presented at EIIC; 1988; Copenhagen, Denmark.

6. Lydahl E, Fagerholm P, Selen G. Implantation of heparin surface modified intraocular lenses in animals. Presented at EIIC; 1988; Copenhagen, Denmark.

7. Steinkogler, FJ, Huber E, Huber-Spitzy V, Aichmair M. Experience with the heparin-modified IOL. Ocular Surgery News. Vol. 8, No. 8.

8. McKoy V. Atomic Force Microscopy of Surface-Passivated IOLs. Presented at the American Society of Cataract and Refractive Surgery's Symposium, 1990; San Francisco, California.

Chapter 11

ROUNDTABLE DISCUSSION WHAT'S NEW IN IOLs

John D. Hunkeler, MD, Moderator

Hunkeler: I'd like to start off this discussion by asking the other members of the panel if they would like to comment about anterior chamber lenses as they stand today? That was not on the list of things that I was going to talk about, but perhaps starting across, would any of the panel members like to talk about anterior chamber lenses? Do you have any comments, Howard?

Gimbel: I think that the verification of accurate placement is as important for anterior chamber lenses as it is for in the bag posterior chamber lenses.

Hunkeler: What do you do in particular in that vein to verify the position of the anterior chamber lens?

Gimbel: I rotate it to position away from the wound, and then I verify the position with the goniolens at surgery.

Hunkeler: With the goniolens?

Gimbel: Yes.

Hunkeler: Cal?

Roberts: The issue comes up in two regards in terms of the choice of a secondary intraocular lens—whether to go with a flexible anterior chamber lens or to go with a fixated posterior chamber lens. I said that as my routine lens, in usual cases, I would use a flexible anterior chamber lens as a secondary IOL in patients who do not have an intact posterior capsule. The second situation which comes up is in corneal transplants. If you are doing either a secondary intraocular lens implantation along with your PK, or whether you are going to do an IOL exchange and there is no intact posterior capsule—are you better off using an anterior chamber lens or to sew in a posterior chamber lens? Now, among the cornea people there is a lot of peer pressure to sew in posterior chamber lenses. This is considered to be more elegant and there is some early data to suggest that this is a better technique. I know from my own series that my results have been better with anterior chamber lenses than they have been with some posterior chamber lenses. So, I think that after having gone through this fad of sewing in posterior chamber lenses routinely in combination with penetrating keratoplasty, I'm starting to go back in many cases to using flexible anterior chamber lenses with a penetrating keratoplasty.

Hunkeler: Let me comment and respond to that very quickly. Roger Steiner at the Academy last year showed equivalent results with sutured-in posterior chamber lenses and anterior chamber lenses. Equivalent results. My most recent experience is in watching Dr. Dhurry suture into the iris a significant number of posterior chamber lenses, at the time of keratoplasty. He claims very good results. I think there is also a recent study just within the last few weeks—Frank Price has much better visual results with sutured-in posterior chamber lenses. I agree, perhaps, with what David Apple said. The answer is not in yet and it is a new technology and new way, but we should be able to get enough experience together to draw a conclusion. Maybe it will turn out that we have equivalent results. Hal?

Balyeat: The bias surgically of anterior segment people, particularly of the keratoplasty doctors, is to keep the lens as far away from the precious cornea as they can. It never did seem to make much sense to me to sew it into the iris, but I think David Apple's work and others' have shown that this is a good technique and it doesn't create the type of iritis and eventual break-down that you would expect. I think, as I said earlier, that the new generation of anterior chamber lenses certainly represents a different lens than we used to have, but occasionally that kind of thinking comes back to haunt us. I am still very concerned about the young people who may have to have secondary implantation and for that reason would favor a transscleral fixation of some type of posterior chamber lens. Of course, the question is where is the cut-off when 60 year olds are physiologically 80 and some are physiologically 40? So, there is a great deal of variation in that. But, I would prefer in the younger patient to use some type of posterior chamber lens.

Apple: John, can I ask you and the panel what you think about the European experience of using these lenses in the anterior chamber in phakic eyes for myopic correction? That's very active over there now; it's been going for maybe nine months to a year with presumed success. Do you think that's crazy?

Hunkeler: I wouldn't call it crazy but I would say I have some questions about it. It was interesting to listen to George Bycoff talk about his results. He has a very significant number of patients with edge glare and fibrosis in the angle with peaking of the pupil and, if you have edge glare with the posterior chamber lenses with the peaking of the pupil in a phakic eye with an anterior chamber lens implant, I think you are really going to have trouble as time goes on down the line and the fibrosis extends at the junction between the foot plate and the haptic and the anterior surface of the iris. I think that is going to be a significant problem. He is reporting 10% peaking of pupils and edge glare at the end of a year. They've got experience well out over a year; it's close to a couple of years. That's my comment. The cornea may tolerate it but I think the symptoms from the relatively small optic that they are dealing with to give enough clearance is going to be a problem.

Hunkeler: Any other comments?

Balyeat: This reminds me a little bit about what's going on right now in terms of doing lensoctomies in high myopes. I think that certainly the initial results might look promising and you have those patients who are terribly gratified, but these patients with high myopia have a pathological eye. Those individuals are subject to glaucoma at a much higher rate, etc. If you have an anterior chamber lens in that eye, many of these patients down the line—even with initial good results— are going to get into very serious trouble just as many patients are going to get into trouble who have had lensectomies for high myopia.

Hunkeler: OK. Why don't we move on to something else. I would like to cover a series of ideas and different concepts that are available today as far as small incisions are concerned. I'll try to get the panel to talk a little bit about the options that we have for smaller incision lens implantation. Henry Clayman came up with the idea of a 5 × 6 mm lens, and there is a more modern version (Figure 11-1), a one-piece PMMA instead of a three-piece, and is a fairly rigid IOL. I could tell you that if you had that little radial tear that is just beginning on the posterior surface and you put a fairly rigid one-piece PMMA lens in, that it is going to most likely tear. So, you have to maybe select a softer configuration in a three-piece 5 × 6 mm lens for that application. Charles Kelman's Phaco-fit lens (Figure 11-2) has an opaque wing and a clear PMMA optic in the center with prolene haptics which actually squeezes down and goes through right around a 4 mm incision (Figure 11-3). The oval 5–6 mm lens goes within a 5 mm incision, allowing for a little bit of stretch. Right now, I don't know where the Alcon project is; I think it is on hold. The Alcon Iogel lens (Figure 11-4) was initially inserted by flat insertion through a 6 mm incision, but the intention was to devise some kind of folding system to put the Iogel lens in. In contradistinction to that is the silicone material of AMO's first generation silicone lens, the SI-18B (Figure 11-5) with an index refraction of 1.41. This lens style has received FDA approval and can be folded

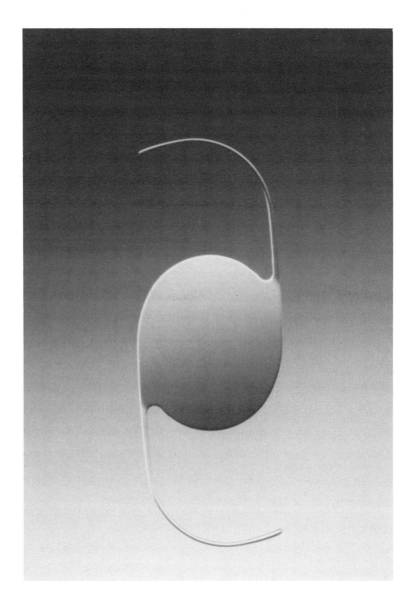

Figure 11-1:   5x6 mm IOPTEX UP-350

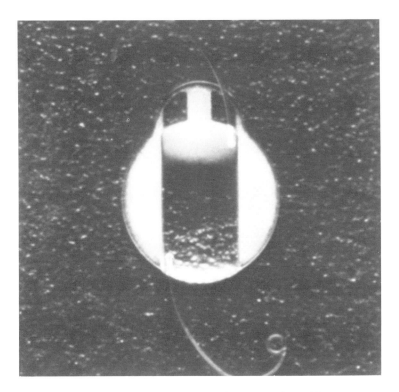

Figure 11-2:   Unfolded Kelman phaco fit PC-28 (AMO)

(Figure 11-6) with a phaco-folder instrument, or Faulkner forceps. More recent is the prodigy system—a mylar sheet that pulls the optic and haptic into a metal tubular injection device. This tube is inserted into the eye, the implant extruded from the tip, then the tube retracted from the eye. I'll also mention the hydrogel lens (Figure 11-7)—the expansile hydrogel—which is also currently on hold for clinical investigation by 3M. This is a dehydrated hydrogel lens that literally expands up to its normal state within a couple of hours (Figure 11-8). There is a newer modified C-loop configuration that seems to work well, and in 24 hours its up to full size (Figure 11-9). The last I would mention is the ORC Memory lens which when heated will go into a new configuration (Figure 11-10), and then you can chill it at that new shape, insert it into the posterior chamber within the capsular bag, and then it expands back within 11 minutes to its normal shape (Figure 11-11). We have a whole myriad of lens implant options. What I would like to ask the panel is where do you feel that things are with the small incision lens implants, and where are you today with the utilization of small incision lens implants? Cal, do you want to start?

Roberts: Yes, because I've learned a lot from a patient of mine. This has not been reported or discussed previously. This was a patient who had been operated in one eye with a conventional 6mm no-holes, J-loop

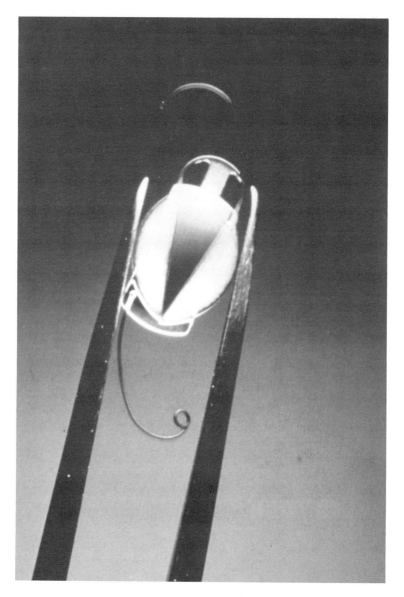

Figure 11-3: Folded Kelman Phacofit PC-28 (AMO)

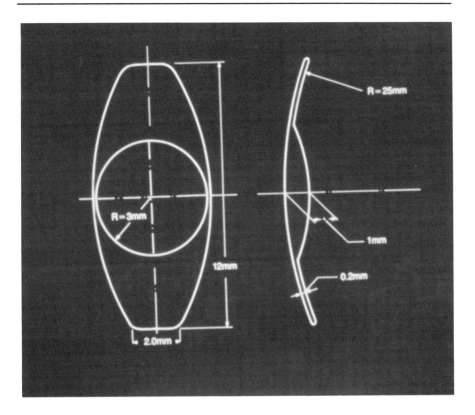

Figure 11-4: ALCON logel lens

style intraocular lens. In the other eye he had one of the Phaco-fit lenses that is the thin, cylindrical looking one with the opaque wings. He came to see me after not getting satisfaction on the fact that he was having so much more glare in the eye with the Phaco-fit lens. He subsequently had three YAG capsulectomies done by his doctor to try to correct for the glare, none of which made any difference. He finally came for another opinion. The lens was placed perfectly and sewn in perfectly, it wasn't a question of that. But, he could actually draw for you where the glare was. You could see the insertion of the wings into the lens when he would draw you an image. You could also see where the wings hinge. It was extraordinarily accurate how well he described the problem with the intraocular lens, when you looked at it sitting in his eye. What I tried doing for him was have him put some Pilo in his eye every morning which helped him with his glare. He did not consider that to be a satisfactory result and, to make a long story short, I explanted the lens and put in a conventional lens to match his other eye after which he complained of no further glare. So, this was a patient with different styles in each eye and he could absolutely see a difference. That has made me suspect the whole idea of small lenses.

Hunkeler: Howard?

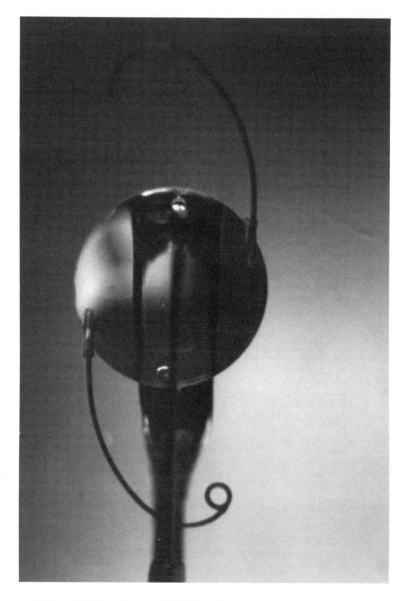

Figure 11-5:   AMO silicone SI-18B unfolded

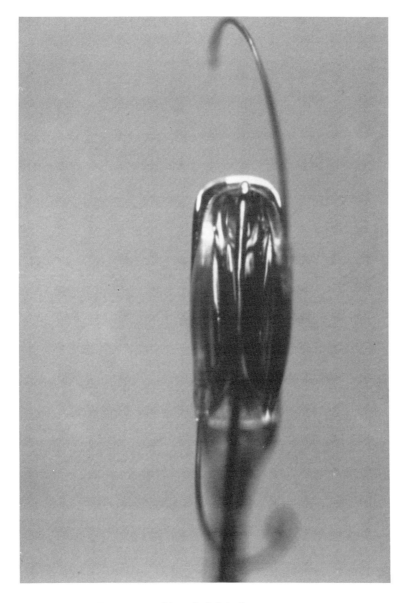

Figure 11-6:   AMO silicone SI-18B folded

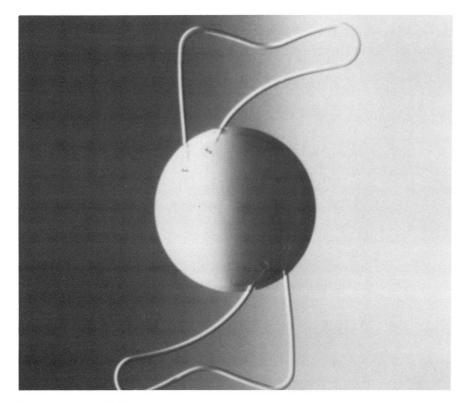

Figure 11-7:   3M hydrogel dehydrated

Gimbel: Speaking about drawing, I would like to just tell you about a patient who illustrates the other end of the spectrum. About a year ago I was convinced I should be using more of the larger optic lenses and go to the one-piece designs, and I had this commercial artist from the paleontology museum in our province come for surgery. He was a young man in his 40's, and I wanted to make sure he had the optimum lens. I put in a 7mm one-piece lens. A couple days after surgery he called me and complained about this crescent in his peripheral vision. I thought that, well, he had the right lens and also in the bag with the capsulorhexis intact, and this couldn't be edge glare. So I thought he had a detachment or something. I brought him in and looked straight on with a slit lamp. I couldn't even see the edge of the lens, and there was no detachment. Everything looked perfect. But, he came with his drawing. He drew just what he saw and that looked like a quarter of the moon, just a crescent. He said that he could see this under varying lighting conditions. So, I had him look a little to one side and then the other and with the direct ophthalmoscope I could see more pink reflex beside the lens on the side opposite to where he saw the crescent of light. Sure enough, it was just so deeply set in his eye that even with a 7mm optic, he could see the edge of the lens and it was not really

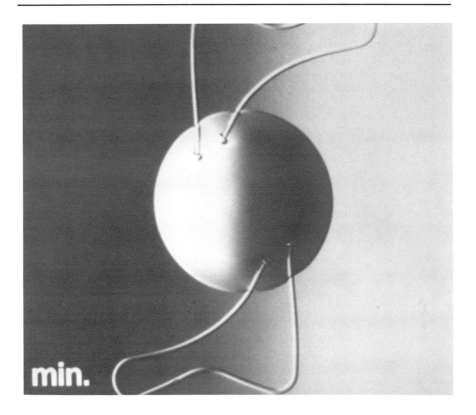

Figure 11-8:   3M hydrogel hydrated at 20 minutes

decentered. It was just maybe 0.5mm off-center as you looked at it. So, I took him back to surgery and I nudged the lens around through the paracentesis until I couldn't center it any better. So, I nudged it to where the lens, if anything, was slightly superior nasally so that if there was any exposed edge inferior temporally, it would be shadowed by the nose and brow. In this case, it convinced me that the 7mm optic does not solve the problem with lens edge glare, and I think that also the vaulting of these long one-piece PMMA lenses is so much more severe.

Hunkeler: You mean the posterior angulation, posterior positioning.

Gimbel: I mean that a 10 degree angulation on a one-piece will vault the lens a lot farther back than on the three-piece.

Hunkeler: I would wonder if that would go away with a period of time. I've had patients complain of that and the symptoms seem to go away of their own accord without doing anything surgically. But, since you did the operation I will assume that that was the cure. Any other comments about small incision lenses?

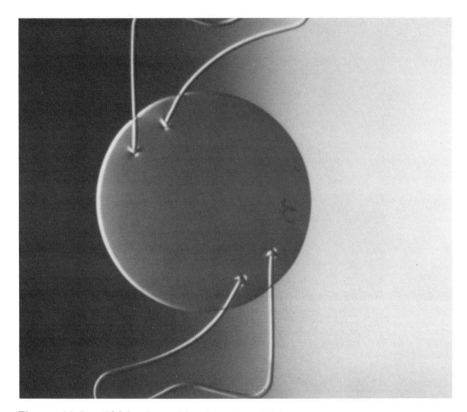

Figure 11-9: 3M hydrogel hydrated at 24 hours

Balyeat: Now that we've had two people present two series of slightly less than 100 patients describing both ends of the spectrum, I'm sure that everybody feels comfortable. I have been using the ovoid lenses, and it just seems to me a natural progression in the things we are doing—that is, phacoemulsification, capsulorhexis, etc.—to be using some kind of smaller lens and being a little bit concerned about some of the properties of the newer materials just primarily because of a lack of experience. The PMMA ovoid lenses seem to be a natural progression. With the first few I put in, I was certainly concerned about seeing patients with edge problems, etc., but that hasn't been the case. I think, again, it gets back to what we've been talking about—capsulotomies.

Hunkeler: You mean about the proper centration with the capsulorhexis.

Balyeat: That's correct, and with a 5mm optic . . . .

Hunkeler: Has it been in your experience, and those others on the panel, that the minimal dimension of the lens is about what you can get the implant through that size incision? So, if it's a 5mm lens you don't

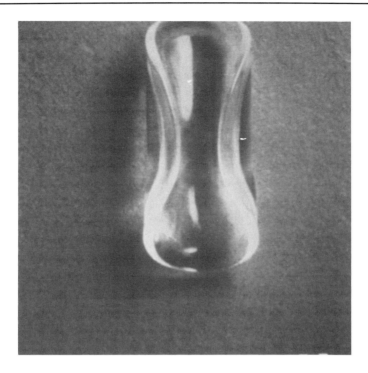

Figure 11-10:   ORC memory lens folded

have to have a 5.5mm incision, and that a 5mm incision will accommodate a 5mm lens, and a 4mm for the foldable lens. Any experience different than that? David, you were going to say something.

Apple: I have a couple of very brief comments about a couple of lenses. The first one relates to the 5 × 6mm. I think when you have younger patients you might have a danger of the problem we already mentioned of having an edge in the pupil. Also with a lens like that—you mentioned that it's very rigid—this lens here if it were 14mm like the standard lens would make the capsular bag like a cigar. I just want to make that comment because of rigidity. So, this goes to the whole point of the new thinking about making lenses a smaller diameter—the 12.5mm or even less—that Dr. Gimbel is involved in. Can we go to the Iogel lens so I can make a comment on those? I think the problem with that lens and also the original Star lens—well, there are two things. One, they were trying to put rectangles into circles. That was a major design problem. These designs may be disappearing. I think one of the reasons they're disappearing is that the design is just too long. It's a 12mm lens. When you look at these in the cadaver eye from behind, the ends of that lens look like tips of skis that are bent up. That lens is way too long. The 12mm lens now is gone; the FDA has taken it away and knows it's too long. The only ones who are going to have a chance of possibly succeeding are the 10 or 11mm length design

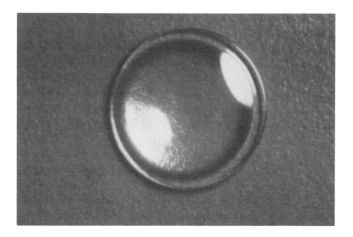

Figure 11-11: ORC memory lens unfolded after 11 minutes

to that lens. It's a nice lens, but the design has to be more appropriate. The shorter the overall length, the more it approaches being a disc. So, that's the thing we have to look at now with the Iogel lens.

Hunkeler: You mentioned that it's a disappearing lens. Unfortunately, that's what happened clinically with enough of these developing total dislocation into the vitreous following YAG laser capsulotomy. Usually, when it occurred early in the postoperative period and relatively early within a few months after the initial surgery, the YAG laser capsulotomy was performed and the tear extended and the Iogel dislocated into the vitreous. I was at a recent meeting where this was discussed and Alcon said four had been dislocated, but there were enough people there at the meeting to account for more than four. So, it sounds like they didn't have all the right numbers.

Apple: I think those lenses are too long and make the capsule too taut. Probably he YAGed them and the thing just split open . . .

Hunkeler: Plus, there is no haptic portion here to be encapsulated by the posterior and anterior capsular collapse.

Apple: The fact that the lens is so biocompatible that it doesn't make an inflammatory response to make a scar to lock it in.

Hunkeler: That's right.

Apple: A lot of problems there.

Gimbel: Could I make one more comment just briefly? I think we need to size the lens to the pupil. Why should we use a 7mm lens if we have done a phaco through a 3mm pupil? I think some pupils are 9mm and others are 3mm at the end of phaco or in a natural state.

Hunkeler: One of my opinions with the smaller pupils is that sometimes you don't know exactly where the capsular bag is when you're finished. You may have a radial tear that is hard to find. I'm a little more concerned about those and may want to go to a little larger optic. Let me slip ahead and we'll talk a little bit about multifocal and bifocal lenses. IOLAB has a multifocal and AMO is beginning a study with their multifocals which have several transitions zones in the optic. Those clinical studies are just beginning. One of the first 3M multifocals I did, I hadn't used the Style-30 implant for a long time. This is the first one of the 3M multifocals that ended up being decentered by 1mm and, in spite of that, it seemed to work very well. So, with that in mind, what comments could we add to what Howard had to say? I would like for him to amplify a little bit perhaps on the symptoms that patients had with this testing about glare and unwanted images. You did report a fairly significant number of patients with some complaints.

Gimbel: It's very interesting how this complaint will vary from patient to patient. In thinking about this, I think it's somewhat analogous to some people being able to tolerate a graduated bifocal and others not. And some people can't even tolerate a bifocal at all, but need two separate pair of glasses and so forth. So, I don't think we will be able to please everybody with the lens, because that symptom may be just too much for some people to adjust to, adapt to, or accept. I think we have to really think about informed consent when it comes to these lenses. As you saw on the film, the majority response is "yes, it's there [glare] but it doesn't bother me that much."

Hunkeler: I would suppose that the potential acid test of all those patients who had their first eye done with a multifocal—that is a 3M multifocal—how many of those would not want one in their other eye? How many would ask to have that implant removed?

Gimbel: We've had no one ask to have it removed. In fact, I've even put the question to those who do seem to not accept it and complain a bit about the glare at night. I even asked them if, now experiencing this, would they rather not have had this lens and put up with bifocals and so forth. They immediately denied that, saying they could tolerate this for the benefit it is giving them. No one asked me to remove it.

Hunkeler: Have you surmised if any of those patients who had their first eye done with the multifocal eye, will put off having the second eye done because of the symptoms?

Gimbel: No.

Hunkeler: So, from your analysis, you don't think it is a clinically significant problem? Well, it's a limited significant clinical problem.

Gimbel: Answering these questions still reflects my careful selection of patients.

Hunkeler: Not using it across the board?

Gimbel: If I used it across the board, I probably would have more people complaining about it. I have recommended against it for young people who have a driving profession and who are out a lot at night or who have any misgivings about some problem with night vision. If so, we decided not to use it.

Roberts: How about the patients who do a lot of reading? Have you compared the best corrected visual acuity of people with conventional monofocal lenses with their reading glasses, to the vision of the bifocal? If you have somebody who reads charts all day long, would you prefer that they had a monofocal IOL with reading glasses or a bifocal IOL?

Gimbel: I think there is a sacrifice—a slight sacrifice—just like bifocals aren't as good as reading glasses and graduated bifocals aren't as good as the line bifocals. I don't think we should tell patients it's going to be just as good. I tell them there is a bit of a trade-off, a little loss of contrast and they may need brighter light, but I still have accountants who elect to have this lens and they are not coming back saying they wish they hadn't.

Hunkeler: I think that has been pretty much the experience—that the quality of vision at near when fully corrected seems to be comparable, and there are a fair number of these patients who have a monofocal IOL in one eye, wearing a bifocal, and the other eye not requiring any add whatsoever. Somehow the images fuse and there is no image size disparity.

Roberts: In patients who have a residual refractive error after having a multifocal lens, are the types of glasses they wear single correction lenses?

Hunkeler: Yes they are.

Roberts: They wear them for distance and near correction equally well?

Gimbel: I was just going to say that I think they are more disappointed— rather than the quality of the vision, I've had a few patients a little disappointed as to the near focal point. In fact, my wife's uncle on whom we did bilateral implants, drifted a little myopic to $-1D$ or so, but he was just annoyed by that focal point being too close. So, he wears his distance correction with an add, an add for the distance focal point which gives him the proper reading distance. So, you can get around it just by using a bifocal.

Hunkeler: Part of the real challenge I think is going to be in our power selection, not only for the distance but the near and getting rid of the cylinder. With this type of multifocal IOL, I think we really are being challenged to the limits of what we can do with our surgery. Any other comments about multifocals? Hal, do you have anything new on IOLs?

Balyeat: No.

Hunkeler: Howard?

Gimbel: In addition to what I just said, I am now tending to, if anything, err on the plus side. Something you have to get over is always aiming for an error on the minus side if anything. I think they are happier if they are plus 0.75 rather than minus 0.75.

Hunkeler: One other thing is the teledioptric system. I think Herb Kaufman and Gholam Peyman at L.S.U. have experience with a teledioptric system for macular degeneration. Apparently, the glasses haven't been worked out perfectly, but it sure is a nice idea to do something for patients with macular degeneration who otherwise might not be helped with cataract surgery. Thank you.

Chapter 12

SECONDARY LENS IMPLANTATION

Hal D. Balyeat, MD

It has been six years since this Symposium has dealt with the subject of secondary lens implantation. Since then much has changed. With conversion to some form of extracapsular surgery ophthalmologists are seeing fewer and fewer aphakic patients without residual capsule. Many of these patients underwent surgery for congenital or young adult onset cataract at a time when intraocular lens implantation was considered unwise in individuals in this age range. These patients have worn contact lenses for many years but have eventually become contact lens failures. Because of an increased incidence of capsular opacification in this age group, many eyes have had primary surgical capsulotomies or subsequent YAG laser capsulotomies. The method of surgical intervention and the type of IOL used will be determined by the presence or absence of adequate capsular support and by the presence or absence of vitreous in the anterior chamber. A thorough preoperative evaluation, including inspection of the chamber angle by gonioscopy, and careful evaluation of the peripheral retina is essential in making this determination. Pachymetry and endothelial cell counts may also be necessary. There are basically four categories of potential candidate eyes for secondary lens implant:

I. Adequate capsular support with intact posterior capsule or capsulotomy without vitreous in the anterior chamber.

   The surgical technique in these eyes involves a superior limbal incision of 6.5 mm to 7.0 mm followed by the introduction of a viscoelastic into the anterior chamber and insertion of a posterior chamber lens into the ciliary sulcus. If the posterior capsule is intact, pre or post lens insertion polishing or post lens insertion capsulotomy may be indicated. If a capsulotomy is present the use of a viscoelastic is usually enough to hold the vitreous behind the capsule. A lens glide is sometimes helpful in positioning the haptics in the sulcus inferiorly.

   If adhesions are present from the posterior surface of the iris to the capsule, these may have to be broken by gentle, blunt or sharp dissection. Extreme care must be used in this maneuver because of the possibility of bleeding. A posterior chamber lens with relatively broad loop haptics is preferred for stability, however, these lenses are more difficult to place if synechia are present. The use of a J loop lens may be indicated if total separation of iris-capsule adhesions is impossible, but the chance of dislocation into the vitreous is increased.

II. Adequate capsular support with vitreous in the anterior chamber.

The primary difference in the surgical technique in this group compared to Group I is the need for anterior vitrectomy prior to posterior lens insertion. Vitrectomy may be performed through the limbal wound or through the pars plana. The surgical technique will be discussed in detail below.

III. Inadequate or absent capsular support without vitreous in anterior chamber.

The primary consideration is whether to use an anterior chamber lens or to suture a posterior chamber lens to the eye wall through the ciliary sulcus. Based on best available information, one assumes that the implantation of a three or four point semi-flexible anterior chamber lens in an older patient with an otherwise normal eye is safe. Past history, however, has taught us that many anterior chamber lenses initially thought to be safe have caused significant complications over time. Will these more recent lens designs stand the test of time? This question is of great importance in decision making concerning lens type and method of implantation. If one believes the more recent lens designs are safe, then should they be implanted in patients of any age requiring secondary lens implantation and if not, what is the appropriate age? Unfortunately, only time will allow us to answer these questions. In the meantime, we will have to use our best clinical judgment in dealing with these problems.

Anterior chamber lens implantation should be performed through a 6.5 mm to 7.0 mm incision approximately 1 mm posterior to the surgical limbus. After entering the anterior chamber, acetylcholine is injected to constrict the pupil. Preoperative miotics may be utilized also. Following pupillary constriction, a viscoelastic is introduced followed by a lens glide. The intraocular lens is inserted as the glide is withdrawn. After positioning of the superior haptics in the chamber angle, the lens is usually rotated clockwise toward the horizontal meridian. This allows the surgeon to evaluate and manipulate the haptics to prevent peripheral iris entrapment. It is also important to position the feet away from any existing peripheral iridectomies. The viscoelastic should be removed partially to prevent the possibility of postoperative elevation of pressure. It is sometimes necessary to leave viscoelastic in order to prevent internal iris prolapse. This condition may also be prevented by performing a peripheral iridectomy if one is not present. Posterior chamber lens implantation in the ciliary sulcus secured by suture fixation to the eye wall has been described by many authors.[1-4] The technique of iris fixation of posterior chamber lenses has been used by corneal transplant surgeons as a means of stabilization. If one is concerned about the long term effects of anterior chamber lenses on the endothelium, then one of the various suture techniques is an alternative.

However, these techniques are not without complications, one of which is endophthalmitis, as noted by Rowsey and Terry (personal communication, January 1990). I favor a variation of the technique described by Lindquist et al:[4] A peritomy is performed superiorly with the addition of two small peritomies at 3 and 9 o'clock. A superior limbal 7.0 mm incision is then made. Viscoelastic is instilled into the anterior chamber. A 10–0 poly-propylene suture on a double armed Ethicon CIF4 needle is cut in half. Each arm is sutured to the haptic of a broad hoop, one piece, 7.0 mm lens. The needle is passed through the pupillary aperture behind the iris in the 3 o'clock meridian passing the needle through the scleral wall 2 mm posterior to the limbus. (Fig. 12-1) The needle is then passed through the sclera posteriorly for approximately 2 mm and the suture is tied on itself. (Fig. 12-2) Leaving the suture loop intact, an additional pass through the sclera is made posteriorly. The suture is then cut allowing the end to retract into the scleral tunnel. (Fig. 12-3) The other needle is then passed through the eye wall in the 9 o'clock meridian and tied in a similar manner. The viscoelastic is then removed and acetyl-choline is instilled constricting the pupil. The wound is then closed with a running 10–0 prolene or mersilene suture. The temporal and nasal conjunctival peritomies are closed with an absorbable suture.

IV. Inadequate or absent capsular support with vitreous in the anterior chamber.

The complication rate of vitrectomy performed at the time of secondary lens implantation, remains a source of debate because of differences in rates reported by several authors.[5–8] Variations in vitrectomy technique may contribute to this disparity. We reviewed 269 cases of secondary intraocular lens implantation and attempted: a) to determine if surgical manipulation of the vitreous increases the complication rate, and b) to compare results in complications associated with limbus-based and pars plana vitrectomy incision sites.[9]

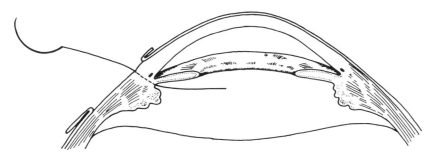

Figure 12-1: The needle is passed through pupillary aperature behind the iris in the 3 o'clock meridian passing the needle through the scleral wall 2 mm posterior to the limbus.

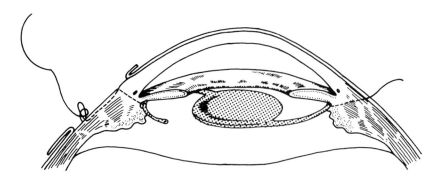

Figure 12-2: The needle is passed through the sclera posteriorly for approximately 2 mm and the suture is tied to itself.

Surgical techniques of secondary IOL implantation were identical except for the performance of a vitrectomy and the surgical location through which the vitrectomy probe was introduced.

All aphakic eyes undergoing secondary lens implantation and followed for at least six months were evaluated for the purposes of this study. Secondary lens implantation was performed in 269 cases and a vitrectomy was performed in 93 (35%) of these cases. A vitrectomy probe was introduced through a limbal incision in 51 cases, and a pars plana incision was employed in the remaining 42.

Surgical techniques were similar in all eyes after all vitreous has been removed from the anterior chamber. The major variables, therefore, were: a) vitrectomy performed at the time of the IOL implantation and b) the incision site which was used for this procedure.

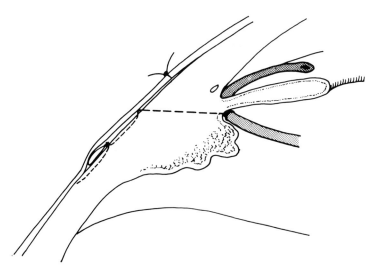

Figure 12-3: The suture is cut allowing the end to retract into the scleral tunnel.

LIMBUS-BASED VITRECTOMY

After completion of a partial thickness limbal incision, the vitrectomy probe and a separate infusion needle are introduced into the anterior chamber. Neither miotics or mydriatics are used preoperatively if a vitrectomy is planned. After removal of the vitreous gel from the anterior chamber, acetylcholine is instilled into the anterior chamber followed by a viscoelastic. The implant is then carried out as previously described.

Pars Plana Vitrectomy

Following the creation of a 6.5 mm limbal groove partial thickness incision, the sclera is cauterized 3.5 mm posterior to the limbus superiorly. A myringotomy knife is then used to perforate the sclera, and the blade tip is visualized through the pupil. The anterior chamber is then entered at the left end of the cornea-scleral grooved incision. The vitrectomy probe is then placed through the pars plana incision, and a 23 gauge infusion needle is placed into the anterior chamber via the limbal wound. (Fig. 12-4) Vitreous is removed from the anterior chamber. The scleral wound is closed with 10–0 nylon. A viscoelastic substance is instilled into the anterior chamber, and the procedure is completed as previously described.

Significant intraoperative complications were not encountered in any of the 269 cases. Postoperatively, visual results were generally good. A

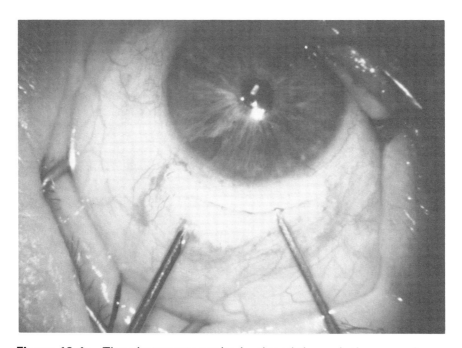

Figure 12-4:   The vitrectomy probe is placed through the pars plana incision, and a 23 gauge infusion needle is placed into the anterior chamber via the limbal wound.

loss of visual acuity of two lines or more on the Snellen chart occurred in 16 (5.9%) cases. In three of the 16 eyes, the visual loss was due to optic nerve or macular problems which appear to be unrelated to the surgical procedure. In the remaining 13 cases, visual acuity loss may have occurred as a complication of surgery. (Table 12-1) Clinical cystoid macular edema was the most common complication occurring in five (2%) of the 269 cases. This occurred in two (2%) of the 93 eyes in which vitrectomy had been performed and 3 (2%) of the 176 eyes in which manipulation of the vitreous was not required. There was no significant difference encountered when vitrectomy incision sites were compared. Retinal detachment occurred in 3 (1%) of 269 cases, none of which occurred in eyes undergoing vitrectomy. Postoperative corneal decompensation occurred in 3 (1%) of the 269 eyes. The incidence was essentially the same in vitrectomized and non-vitrectomized cases. The postoperative endophthalmitis occurred in a single case in which a vitrectomy was not performed, and significant postoperative glaucoma, associated with vitreous loss, was observed in a single eye following a vitrectomy and secondary lens implant.

Previous authors have reported complication rates following secondary lens implantation with or without vitrectomy, and these problems have occurred in from 5.3% to 10% of cases. These previous reports have suggested that aphakic eyes with vitreous in the anterior chamber have a significantly higher complication rate than those in which vitreous gel remains behind the iris plane. Complications of surgery include cystoid macular edema, retinal detachment, corneal decompensation, and pupillary distortion.

This study did not demonstrate an increased complication rate associated with closed mechanical anterior vitrectomy through the limbus-based or pars plana incision site.

Although unplanned vitreous loss occurring at the time of cataract extraction is clearly associated with an increased incidence of postoper-

Table 12-1: Eyes suffering loss of two or more Snellen lines of visual acuity.

PROBLEM	# EYES
Clinical CME	5
Retinal Detachment	3
Bullous Keratopathy	3
Endophthalmitis	1
Glaucoma	1
Macular Degeneration	2
Ischemic Optic Neuropathy	1

ative complications, planned limited anterior vitrectomy, performed in a "closed eye" situation, may be associated with a much lower incidence of problems following secondary intraocular lens implantation. Although a pars plana incision site is usually preferred for posterior closed vitrectomy techniques, this study demonstrates that a limbal approach is as safe and effective as a pars plana site for the performance of a limited anterior vitrectomy. At this time we, nevertheless, favor the pars plana approach because of the probability that it is associated with less endothelial cell damage.

Special Considerations in Secondary Lens Implantation Technique

I. Wound Location

Decision making concerning wound location is multi-factorial. Previous wound location is an important consideration. Prior peritomy usually results in conjunctival scarring and recession making a standard peritomy difficult. Frequently, light cautery along the length of the proposed incision at, or behind the surgical limbus, is sufficient in barring the sclera. Entering the eye at the site of the previous incision is not contraindicated. Residual suture remnants may have to be removed at the time of the incision. If an inadvertent filtering bleb exists, and especially if wound separation and "against the rule" astigmatism is present, entering through the previous wound is helpful. However, the incision should be made away from, or in front of, a filtering bleb used for glaucoma control. Incisions in the horizontal meridian are technically more difficult and should be reserved for eyes with excessive "with the rule" cylinder or in eyes with peripheral iris synechia or large iridectomies if a decision has been made preoperatively not to lyse the synechia or repair the iridectomy.

II. Iris

Peripheral iridectomies are usually present adjacent to the incision site. Oftentimes, vitreous presents spontaneously through these openings immediately after the incision or following lens insertion prior to wound closure. Introducing the vitrectomy instrument through the pars plana is helpful in removal of the vitreous underlying the peripheral iridectomy site. If vitreous presents through the iridectomy site at the completion of lens insertion, removal with an automated vitrectomy instrument or cellulose sponges followed by the introduction of a viscoelastic or air into the anterior chamber is indicated to prevent vitreous adhesion to the wound.

One of the most common causes of lens dislocation following secondary implantation of an anterior chamber intraocular lens is dislocation of a haptic through the peripheral iridectomy site superiorly. (Fig. 12-5) This causes a relative shortening of the diameter of the lens resulting in migration of the inferior haptics toward the endothelium. It is important to rotate the lens haptics toward the horizontal meridians to prevent migration into the peripheral iridectomy site. Rotation of the haptics may lead to iris entrapment by the foot plates. This, in turn, may lead to pupillary elongation and endothelial loss overlying the haptic. It is important to make sure the iris is not trapped by the haptic. This can be accomplished by using a hook to bring the feet away from the angle and simultaneously evaluate the appearance of the pupil. Anterior chamber lenses with positioning holes at the edge of the optic may be helpful in this maneuver.

Another common problem which may be encountered is internal iris prolapse. This may occur during the procedure, following wound closure, or postoperatively. This commonly occurs in older eyes with blue irides. Intraoperative iris prolapse with loss of iris pigment, preoperative mydriatics or the use of intraoperative epinephrine will accentuate this problem. Frequently, it is not apparent until the viscoelastic is removed at the completion of the procedure. It occurs in the postoperative state after pupillary dilation, either physiologic or when induced pharmacologically. Internal iris prolapse may be prevented in the intraoperative state by: a) pupillary constriction with intraoperative miotics; b) performing a peripheral iridectomy at the site of the prolapse or adjacent to it and/or; c) leaving the viscoelastic material in the anterior chamber. When internal iris prolapse occurs postoperatively, it is sometimes successfully treated by either dilation or pupillary constriction. Occasionally laser iridotomy is necessary. This condition can be differentiated from pupillary block glaucoma by intraocular pressure determination.

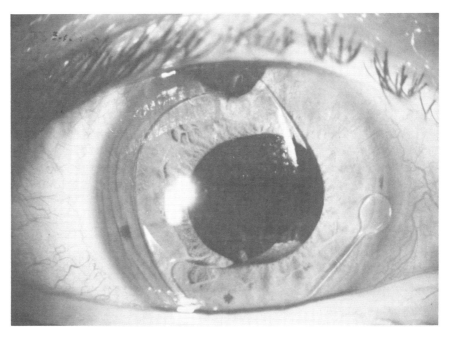

Figure 12-5:   Dislocation of a haptic through the peripheral iridectomy site superiorly.

III. Residual Posterior Capsule

If the posterior capsule is intact, one should consider polishing the capsule at the time of posterior chamber lens implantation. This is especially appropriate when dealing with eyes at risk such as high myopia or patients with CME or retinal detachment in the fellow eye after uneventful surgery. If a capsulotomy is indicated, it can be carried out at the completion of the procedure using a cystotome or bent needle.

Often times, the patient has had a primary or secondary capsulotomy but enough capsule remains to implant a posterior chamber lens without the need for suture fixation. If posterior synechiae to the capsule do not exist, implantation is carried out in the usual manner. A broad loop lens is indicated because it provides increased contact with the sulcus. Also, J loop lenses have a tendency to rotate in an anterior-posterior direction if capsular support is inadequate. Oftentimes, however, synechiae are present preventing easy insertion of the haptics into the ciliary sulcus. These synechiae may be lysed by sharp dissection with 11 mm Vannas scissors under a viscoelastic.[10] Adhesions may also be broken with an iris spatula. Bleeding from the iris is common but can usually be controlled by increasing the intraocular pressure mechanically with the introduction of more viscoelastic. If two opposite quadrants can be freed of adhesions, a J loop lens may be inserted. It is important, however, that adequate capsule exists, otherwise the lens may dislocate into the vitreous. Based on past experience, it is preferable to use transscleral fixation if one is unable to free the adhesions enough to allow for the insertion of a broad loop lens. Disinsertion of the capsule may occur during blunt dissection resulting in postoperative lens dislocation.

Summary

Intraocular lens implantation, both primary and secondary, is continuing to change. New materials and techniques make this inevitable. Today's methods will be obsolete tomorrow. The primary unresolved question of importance is how safe are anterior chamber lenses. If the new designs prove effective in eliminating the major complications which we have seen in the past, the anterior chamber lens will be the lens of choice in most adult eyes. However, until it can be demonstrated that these lenses are safe, posterior chamber lenses should be utilized in all eyes with adequate capsular support and in younger patients without capsular support by suturing the lens to the eye wall. How young is young? Assuming a healthy endothelium, posterior chamber lenses should be used in individuals below the age of sixty. This is, of course, arbitrary. Many individuals below sixty are physiologically much older and vice versa. This must be taken into account. Individuals with a limited life expectancy may be candidates for anterior chamber lenses regardless of age. The newer design anterior chamber lenses may prove to be much safer than previous lens designs, however, it will be many years before this question will be resolved. We may find, on the other hand, that techniques currently used to suture posterior chamber lenses to the eye wall will not stand the test of time due to late occurring complications such as endophthalmitis secondary to suture erosion.

References

1. Malbran ES, Malbran E Jr., Negri I: Lens Guide Suture for Transport and Fixation in Secondary IOL Implantation After Intracapsular Extraction. Int Ophthalmol 1986; 9:151–160.
2. Spigelman AV, Lindstrom RL, Nichols SD, et al: Implantation of a Posterior Chamber Lens Without Capsular Support During Penetrating Keratoplasty or as a Secondary Lens Implant. Ophthalmic Surg 1988; 19:396–398.
3. Stark WJ, Goodman G, Goodman D, Gottsch J: Posterior Chamber Intraocular Lens Implantation in the Absence of Posterior Capsular Support. Ophthalmic Surg 1988; 19:240–243.
4. Lindquist TD, Agapitos PJ, Lindstrom RL, Lane SS, Spigelman AV: Transscleral Fixation of Posterior Chamber Intraocular Lenses in the Absence of Capsular Support. Ophthalmic Surg 1989; 20:769–775.
5. Shammas JF, Milkie CF: Secondary Lens Implantation in Aphakia: Visual Results and Complications: AM Intra-Ocular Implant Soc J 1978; 4:180–183.
6. Lindstrom RL, Harris WS: Secondary Anterior Chamber Lens Implantation: CLAO Journal 1984; 10(2):133–136.
7. Cozean CH: A Longer view of Secondary Intraocular Lens Implantation With Special Emphasis on the Role of the Vitreous. Am Intra-Ocular Implant Soc J 1980; 6:361–362.
8. Wong SK, Koch DD, Emery JM: Secondary Intraocular Lens Implantation. J Cataract Refract Surg 1987; 13:17–20.
9. Balyeat HD, Poley BJ, Wilkinson CP: Secondary Lens Implantation With Vitrectomy. Pars plana or limbal approach? Presented at the ASCRS Symposium on Cataract, IOL and Refractive Surgery: March, 1988; Los Angeles, CA.
10. Dahan E, Salmenson BD, Levin J: Ciliary Sulcus Reconstruction for Posterior Implantation in the Absence of an Intact Posterior Capsule. Ophthalmic Surg 1989; 20:776–780.

Chapter 13

INTRAOCULAR MIOTICS AND THE CORNEAL ENDOTHELIUM

Calvin W. Roberts, MD, Ritsuko Akiyama, MD,
Jan P. Koniarek, PhD, Kunyan Kuang, MD,
Jorge Fischbarg, MD, PhD

Anterior chamber miotic solutions have been used in ocular surgery for more than 25 years and the value of pupillary miosis during cataract extraction, intraocular lens implantation, corneal transplant, glaucoma surgery, anterior vitrectomy, and other anterior segment procedures is well recognized. Pupillary constriction secures the placement of an intraocular lens, protects the crystalline lens during anterior chamber surgery, and prevents incarceration of the peripheral iris in the surgical incision. More recently, their value in controlling intraocular pressure during the first postoperative day has been widely reported.

The two agents available commercially are acetylcholine 1.0% and carbachol (carbaminoylcholine) 0.01%. They differ not only in terms of their onset, intensity and duration of action, but also in terms of ocular and systemic side effects.

Acetylcholine is the naturally occurring neurohumoral transmitter for autonomic ganglia and skeletal muscle (nicotinic action) and for postganglionic parasympathetic nerve fibers (muscarinic action). It is a natural vasodilator, a cardiac depressant, and a stimulant of the vagus nerve and the entire parasympathetic nerve system. The muscarinic actions can be abolished by atropine while the nicotinic actions are blocked by tubocurarine. Acetylcholine in high doses produces coronary vasodilation, decreased myocardial contractility, and bradycardia. Continuous doses of acetylcholine cause cardiac arrest.

In the eye, postganglionic parasympathetic fibers from the ciliary ganglion innervate the sphincter pupillae, causing miosis, and the ciliary muscle, resulting in changes in accomodation and in the facility of outflow. Exogenous acetylcholine administered intracamerally can duplicate some of the effects of parasympathetic stimulation. Amsler and Verrey first established the miotic effect of intracameral acetylcholine in 1949.[1] Barraquer[2] may have been the first to use acetylcholine routinely in anterior segment surgery. Since then, the value of acetylcholine induced miosis has been established for cataract surgery and intraocular lens implantation.

Acetylcholine is rapidly broken down by the action of acetylcholinesterase. Thus it is commonly classified as a short acting miotic.

Carbachol (carbaminoylcholine) is a potent synthetic choline ester, differing from acetylcholine by a carbaminoyl (NH_2CO) group in place of an acetyl (CH_3CO) group attached to the choline base. Its general pharmacologic properties were first described by Kreitmair in 1932.[3] Like acetylcholine, carbachol is primarily a direct-acting agent, with muscarinic and nicotine effects. It may also cause the release of endogenous acetylcholine from cholinergic nerve fiber terminals or partially inhibit cholinesterase. It has an inhibitory effect on secretion by the ciliary body. Because carbachol is resistant to hydrolysis by cholinesterase, it is active for much longer than acetylcholine. On a weight basis, it is 100 times more potent than acetylcholine. Thus commercial preparations are a 0.01% solution compared to 1.0% for acetylcholine.

Topical carbachol has been used as an anti-glaucoma medication for over 50 years. Because the molecule carries a positive charge, it penetrates poorly through the corneal epithelium. Surfactants such as benzalkonium chloride are necessary to increase corneal penetration. In 1965, Reed described the use of intracameral carbachol as an alternative to acetylcholine for intraocular miosis.[4] Subsequent clinical and experimental studies have established that the miotic effect of carbachol is more intense and of longer duration than with acetylcholine.

Systemic effects from intraocular use of acetylcholine are rare. Those reported include hypotension, bradycardia, bronchospasm, and sweating. Systemic effects from carbachol are clinically more common, with patients complaining of brow ache, headache, nausea, abdominal cramps and tightness in the urinary bladder. Corneal clouding, persistent bullous keratopathy and postoperative iritis following cataract extraction with utilization of intraocular carbachol have been occasionally reported.[5]

Recently we have shown that carbachol is also associated with greater postoperative intraocular inflammation that is acetylcholine.[6]

Recent studies have reported changes in the morphology and physiology of the corneal endothelium associated with *in vitro* use of acetylcholine and carbachol. Vaughn, Hull, and Green perfused rabbit corneal endothelial cells for 15 minutes in a specular microscope with either carbachol solution, acetylcholine solution, or balanced salt controls. The acetylcholine solution and the balanced salt controls showed no change in corneal physiology, while the carbachol solution produced abnormal corneal swelling. None of the solutions resulted in any abnormality of morphology.[7]

Yee and Edelhauser repeated these studies using a reformulated carbachol solution and found that there was greater corneal swelling with the commercially prepared carbachol solution than with the commercially prepared acetylcholine solution.[8]

Birnbaum, Hull, Green, and Frey then repeated their earlier studies, this time comparing the carbachol in its commercially prepared BSS vehicle to the identical BSS vehicle without the carbachol. As corneas perfused with the BSS vehicle performed similar to controls, and the corneas perfused with the carbachol containing solution had significantly increased corneal swelling rate, they concluded that carbachol itself was inherently toxic to the endothelium.[9]

Yee then studied the acetylcholine vehicle and determined that it was the lack of an appropriate salt buffer in the commercially prepared solution, and not the acetylcholine or mannitol that was responsible for the abnormal values he had reported earlier.[10] Subsequently, the commercially prepared solution of acetylcholine was reformulated to include NaCl, KCl, MgCl, and $CaCl_2$.

To better understand the effect of acetylcholine and carbachol on the corneal endothelium, and to try to make sense out of these somewhat contradictory reports, we designed a series of experiments to study the active agents separately and in combination with the vehicles present in commercial intraocular solutions.

To understand the effect of drugs on the corneal endothelium, it is necessary to review the physiology of the cornea.

Proper corneal hydration is necessary for corneal clarity. The cornea is clear because the distance between corneal lamellae and the density of water is maintained at a level that allows light to pass through without scattering.[11] If the cornea fills with fluid, its appearance becomes hazy and visual acuity drops precipitously. The mucopolysaccharides within the stroma continuously pull water into the stroma from the anterior chamber. Thus it is the role of the endothelium to actively pump water out of the stroma into the anterior chamber to maintain normal corneal hydration. The corneal pump continuously counteracts the leak of water into the stroma so that a steady-state balance in water flow results.[12]

As the endothelium is unable to actively pump water, this cellular monolayer generates an electrical transendothelial potential difference (TEPD). This TEPD leads to electrolyte transport and movement of fluid by osmosis. Although the exact mechanism of ionic transport in the endothelium is not known, all proposed models of ion flow include the presence of sodium potassium adenosine triphosphatase (Na^+-K^+ATPase) in the lateral cell membrane and bicarbonate (HCO_3) transport from the cell to the aqueous through the apical membrane.[13-16] The net result of this movement of ions is the anterior chamber becoming negative in ionic charge compared to the stroma which can be measured as an electrical potential difference across the endothelium of approximately 0.5mV.[17]

This transendothelial potential difference (TEPD) is a sensitive and predictive indicator of the viability of the corneal endothelial pump. Factors that inhibit the endothelial pump also diminish the TEPD.[18] Thus one technique for assessing the viability of the endothelium and its reaction to miotic solutions is to measure the TEPD while bathing the endothelium with various solutions.

Methods

Three kilogram male New Zealand white rabbits were sacrificed with an overdose of sodium pentobarbital injected into the marginal ear vein and the eyes were enucleated. The corneal epithelium was removed and the corneas mounted in chambers.

The technique and experimental design for measuring TEPD has been described by Fischbarg.[17] This measurement is performed in a two-part chamber, using two calomel electrodes connected by saline bridges to the two sections of the chamber (Figure 13-1). The chamber was enclosed in a Faraday cage to eliminate electromagnetic interference. The experiments were performed at 37 degrees.

The following solutions were selected:
1. Solution A - Carbachol in balanced salt vehicle
2. Solution B - Acetylcholine in mannitol vehicle
3. Solution C - Acetylcholine with some of the mannitol replaced with balanced salts (acetylcholine with electrolytes)
4. Solution D - Same as Solution C, but adding carbachol to make an acetylcholine/carbachol mixture
5. Balanced salt solution (BS) control

The composition of the experimental solutions is given in Table 13-1. BS is a balanced salt solution without sucrose prepared in our laboratory. For pH control, oxygenation, and stirring, the solutions were continuously bubbled with a mixture of 5% CO_2 and 95% air.

Each experiment was begun by taking a control reading of the TEPD with balanced salts BSS bathing both the stromal and the endothelial sides of the preparation. The TEPD was monitored until it stabilized. This provided the baseline value of the TEPD to which all later measurements in a given experiment were compared. At this point, the BSS solution on the endothelial side was replaced by the appropriate exper-

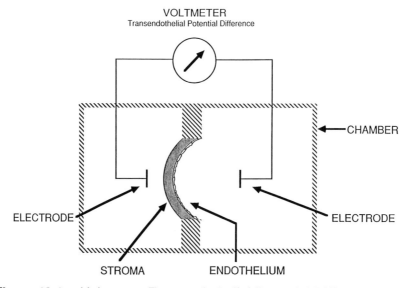

VOLTMETER
Transendothelial Potential Difference

CHAMBER

ELECTRODE

ELECTRODE

STROMA   ENDOTHELIUM

Figure 13-1:   Voltmeter, Transendothelial Potential Difference

Table 13-1:   Ionic composition of miotic solutions (mM/L).

	Balanced salts (BS)	Solution A	Solution B	Solution C	Solution D
NaCl	112.9	109.60	0	5.10	5.10
NaHCO3	39.2	0	0	0	0
KCl	0	10.00	0	5.40	5.40
KHCO3	3.8	0	0	0	0
MgCl	0	1.50	0	1.50	1.50
KH2PO4	1.0	0	0	0	0
MgSO4	0.8	0	0	0	0
CaCl2	1.7	3.25	0	0.70	0.70
AcetCh	0	0	55.05	55.05	55.05
Mannitol	0	0	164.65	153.70	153.70
Carbachol	0	0.55	0	0	0.19
Na acetate	0	28.65	0	0	0
Na citrate	0	5.79	0	0	0
Osmolarity	298	309	290	285	287

imental test solution, and the endothelial side was exposed to it for one hour. Then the test solution was again replaced with BSS on the endothelial side and the TEPD monitored until a steady-state reading was obtained. TEPD was not measured while the test solution was on the endothelial side, since the ionic concentration of the test solution would mask the small TEPD of the endothelium. Only with the identical BSS solution bathing the endothelium at all measurements would the TEPD measurements be accurate.

This cycle of bathing the endothelium with the test solution followed by BSS for TEPD measurement was repeated for as long as the TEPD remained at least 5% of the initial value. If it was less, the experiment was terminated.

Results

The results are shown in Figure 13-2 (taken from Koniarek et al).[19] The solution of acetylcholine with electrolytes maintained the highest TEPD and had the longest experimental life, lasting approximately eight hours. BSS, commercially prepared carbachol, and the acetylcholine/carbachol mixture performed similarly, lasting approximately six hours. The com-

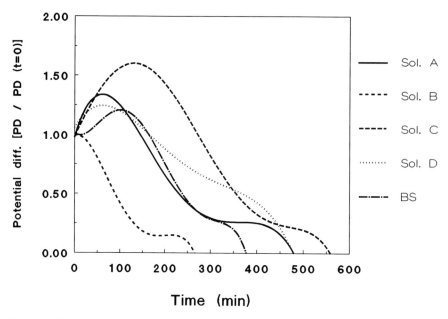

Figure 13-2:   Graphic display of experimental results

mercially prepared acetylcholine without electrolytes performed the worst, with low TEPD and experimental life of only 4 hours.

Discussion

As a small difference in the composition of the acetylcholine vehicle, adding balanced salts, produced dramatic differences in its effect on corneal endothelial physiology, we confirmed the results of Yee et al[10] that balanced salts are necessary to bathe the endothelium. As the only difference between the acetylcholine with electrolytes and the mixed acetylcholine/carbachol solution was the presence of carbachol, and the mixed solution performed poorer than the acetylcholine with electrolytes solution, our study lends supports to the conclusions of Birnbaum et al[9] that carbachol was toxic for the endothelium.

Thus the use of TEPD as the experimental parameter confirms the results obtained by others using rate of corneal swelling, and expands our knowledge to the point where we can account for the apparent discrepancies in the earlier literature. In particular this study serves to emphasize the role of the vehicle solutions in these physiologic measurements.

To further explore the longstanding question as to whether acetylcholine or carbachol by themselves have any effect on the corneal endothelium, we decided to prepare solutions of acetylcholine and carbachol in our laboratory using identical balanced salt solution vehicles for both agents. By testing them in this way, with the same vehicle and with that same balanced salt solution vehicle as the control, the only experimental variable would be the active ingredient.

The composition of the three solutions is listed in Table 13-2. Note that to maintain the solutions isotonic, 59.8 mM/l of NaCl was removed from the acetylcholine solution. All the other constituents were the same.

The procedure here was different from that in the prior experiments described above. Corneas were mounted in Dikstein-Maurice chambers, and corneal thickness was measured with a specular microscope for three hours while the endothelial side of the preparation was perfused at a rate of 1.4 ml/h with the test solution. The de-epithelialized stromal surface of the corneas was covered by silicone oil. Thickness measurements were performed every fifteen minutes. The chamber was maintained in a thermal jacket at 37 degrees C.

The results are presented in Figure 13-3 (taken from Akiyama et al).[20] The rate of corneal swelling is plotted against time for each solution. The rate of corneal swelling in the presence of the carbachol solution was significantly greater than that with either acetylcholine or BSS control. Though the corneal swelling rate is slightly lower with acetylcholine than with control, the difference was not significant.

These results reinforce our findings from the TEPD studies, that acetylcholine appears benign to the corneal endothelium. It is also in line with the results of Birnbaum et al,[9] who measured rates of corneal swelling with the commercially prepared carbachol solution and the identical vehicle without carbachol and found that the carbachol containing solution had a higher swelling rate.

As our study and that of Birnbaum et al[9] had similar results, the conclusion of endothelial toxicity of carbachol becomes more evident. Whereas acetylcholine is a naturally occurring substance that is normally present in the anterior chamber and would be expected to have no adverse effect on the endothelium, carbachol is a synthetic agent.

While no clinical studies on the corneal endothelium have yet identified adverse effects from intraocular carbachol, it should be recognized that

Table 13-2: Composition of concentrations of the three solutions

Solutions	BS	1%Ach	0.01%Carb
NaCl	116.80	57.00	116.8
NaHCO3	39.2	39.2	39.2
KHCO3	3.80	3.80	3.80
KH2PO4	1.00	1.00	1.00
MgSO4	0.78	0.78	0.78
CaCl2(2H2O)	1.70	1.70	1.70
Acetylch.Cl		55.05	
Carbachol Cl			0.55
OSMOLARITY	298.2	298.2	299.2

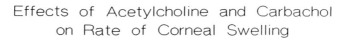

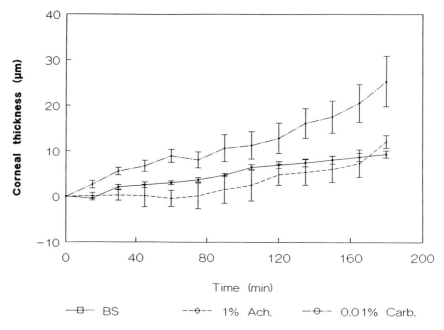

Figure 13-3:   Graphic display of the effects of Acetylcholine and Carbachol on the rate of corneal swelling

the solutions in the anterior chamber at the end of a cataract extraction remain in contact with the endothelium for many hours. Assuming the following fluid capacity:

Anterior chamber	0.250ml
Posterior chamber	0.060ml
Space left by extracted crystalline lens	0.250ml
Subtotal fluid capacity	0.560ml
Posterior chamber IOL	−0.035ml
Total fluid capacity	0.525ml

Assuming a normal aqueous flow rate of approximately 0.002ml/minute, then the minimum time necessary for aqueous replacement is

$$\frac{0.525 \text{ ml}}{0.002\text{ml/min}} = 262.5 \text{ mins. (4 hours, 23 minutes)}$$

Should in fact, the aqueous flow rate be reduced, as is normally seen following intraocular surgery, the solutions left in the anterior chamber at the end of surgery may be present for six or eight hours postop. Thus it is important to have the most physiologic solutions present as possible.

In our study, the increased swelling rate of the corneal endothelium with carbachol was seen from the outset and tended to increase at three hours when the experiment was ended. Clinically, though the aqueous concentration of carbachol will continually decrease as aqueous is produced, it may still be exerting an effect for a much longer time. The effect on the pupil and ciliary body persist for several days. The effect on the corneal endothelium may be similarly prolonged.

Surgeons using intraocular miotics should consider the effect of these agents on the cornea. Compromised endothelium, such as that seen in Fuchs dystrophy or following penetrating keratoplasty may be more at risk, along with any situation in which corneal edema from poorly functioning endothelium is present.

References

1. Amsler M, Verrey F. Mydriase et myose directes en instances par les mediateurs chimiques. Ann Ocul, 1949, 182:936.
2. Barraquer JI. Acetylcholine as a miotic agent for use in surgery. Am J Ophthalmol, 1964, 57:406.
3. Kreitmair H. Eine neue klasse cholinester, Arch Exp. Pathol Pharmakol, 1932, 164:346.
4. Reed H. Use of carbamylcholine chloride. Am J Ophthalmol, 1965, 59:955.
5. Physicians' Desk Reference For Ophthalmology, Oradell, NJ, Medical Economics Co, 17th edition, 1989, p. 83.
6. Roberts CW. Control of cataract extraction postoperative intraocular pressure with intracameral miotics, New Orleans Academy of Ophthalmology, 1990.
7. Vaughn ED, Hull DS, Green K. Effects of intraocular miotics on the corneal endothelium. Arch Ophthalmol, 1978, 96:1897.
8. Yee RW, Edelhauser HF. Comparison of intraocular acetylcholine and carbachol. J Cataract Refract Surg, 1986, 12:18.
9. Birnbaum DB, Hull DS, Green K, Frey NP. Effect of carbachol on rabbit corneal endothelium. Arch Ophthalmol, 1987, 105:253.
10. Yee RW, Wallace G, Yu HS. Effects of the components of Miochol and Miostat on bovine corneal endothelial cells in vitro. Investigative Ophthalmol Vis Sci, 1989 (suppl), 30(3):335.
11. Maurice DM. The cornea and sclera. in *The Eye*, vol 1B, Davson H, ed., Orlando, Acad Press, 1984, p.1–158.
12. Dikstein S, Maurice DM. The metabolic basis of the fluid pump in the cornea. J Physiol, 1972, 221:29–41.
13. Fischbarg, J, Lim JJ. Role of cations, anions, and carbonic anhydrase in fluid transport across rabbit corneal endothelium. J Physiol, 1974, 241:647–75.
14. Fischbarg J, Hofer GL, Koatz RA. Priming the fluid pump by osmotic gradients across rabbit corneal endothelium. Biochim Biophys Acta, 1980, 603:198–206.
15. Fischbarg J, Hernandez J, Liebovitch LS, Koniarek JP. The mechanism of fluid and electrolyte transport across corneal endothelium: critical revision and update of model. Curr Eye Res, 1985, 4:351–60.

16. Hodson S. The regulation of corneal hydration by a salt pump requiring the presence of sodium and bicarbonate ions. J Physiol (Lond), 1974, 236:271–302.

17. Fischbarg J. Potential difference and fluid transport across rabbit corneal endothelium. Biochim Biophys Acta, 1972, 228:362–6.

18. Barfort P, Maurice DM. Electrical potential and fluid transport across the corneal endothelium. Exp Eye Res, 1974, 19:11–19.

19. Koniarek JP, Akiyama R, Roberts CW, Liebovitch LS, Fischbarg J. Anterior chamber miotic solutions: Effects on transendothelial electrical potential difference, in preparation.

20. Akiyama R, Kuang R, Roberts CW, Fischbarg J. Effects of acetylcholine and carbachol on rabbit corneal endothelial function, in preparation.

Chapter 14

CATARACT SURGERY IN ANTICOAGULATED PATIENTS

Calvin W. Roberts, MD, Suzanne M. Woods, RN, BSN
Liebert S. Turner, MD

Abstract

A prospective study was performed on 25 patients undergoing planned extracapsular cataract extraction with posterior chamber intraocular lens implantation who were considered to be anticoagulated on the basis of their medical history or the medicine they were taking. The patients were instructed to continue their usual medications throughout the perioperative period including on the day of surgery. All patients but one had routine narcoleptic sedation and retrobulbar anesthesia. The surgical technique was altered to use an inferior corneal traction suture and a single planed clear corneal incision. No intraoperative or postoperative anterior chamber bleeding was experienced. The observed complications were increased awareness of corneal sutures, increased endothelial cell loss, delayed visual rehabilitation due to with-the-rule astigmatism and transient corneal edema. All patients achieved 20/40 or better visual acuity without corneal edema by three months post-surgery.

As an increasing number of geriatric patients are pharmacologically anticoagulated for cardiovascular or cerebrovascular disease, it is valuable to perform cataract surgery safely without risking complications from temporarily discontinuing these medications.

Introduction

With the increasing number of patients maintained on aspirin or other anticoagulants for cardiac or cerebrovascular disease, the potential exists for significant intraoperative and perioperative hemorrhage during cataract surgery.

Several authors have recommended withholding of anticoagulant preoperatively.[1-4] The experience of others has been that cataract surgery can be performed safely without withholding anticoagulants.[5-8] McMahon[9] and Gainey et al[10] have documented a greater incidence of hyphema in anticoagulated patients compared to non-anticoagulated controls. In a survey of the American Intraocular Implant Society, 75% of surgeons temporarily discontinue warfarin sodium prior to and following surgery and 53% discontinue aspirin.[11]

In the past we have encountered bleeding when the patients were anticoagulated, and medical complications when these medications were discontinued preoperatively. (Case reports)

Thus we have strived to develop a surgical protocol for all patients on anticoagulants or whose medical history suggests the possibility of a bleeding disorder. We report here on a prospective study of twenty-five consecutive cases in whom there was a significant risk for inadequately controllable bleeding associated with surgery.

Case Reports

1. A 70 year old woman underwent extracapsular cataract extraction with intraocular lens implantation on March 26, 1986. Her medical history was significant only for a hiatus hernia and mild osteoarthritis. She claimed to be on no medication when interviewed independently by the attending physician, resident physician, two nurses, and the anesthesiologist. Bipolar cautery was used to obtain hemostasis in the cataract section and the procedure was uneventful.

   On the first post-operative day there was a 100% hyphema, a clear cornea, and intraocular pressure of 25 mm/Hg. The patient was begun on acetazolamide 250 mg QID, and timolol maleate 0.5% BID, in addition to the routine gentamicin and prednisolone acetate 1% drops QID. On review of the history, the patient stated she had taken 300 aspirin tablets in the past month since her husband died because her osteoarthritis had flared up.

   Since she had taken aspirin as recently as the day of surgery, it was elected not to evacuate the hyphema. By the third post-operative day the blood had begun to absorb. Blood staining of the cornea was noted. A clot began to form on the fifth post-operative day.

   The anterior chamber was clear of blood in five weeks. The blood staining resolved in eighteen months. The final visual acuity was 20/100 secondary to an epiretinal membrane.

2. A 79 year old man underwent extracapsular cataract extraction with intraocular lens implantation on April 4, 1988. The patient had Waldenstrom's macroglobulinemia and underwent plasmapheresis every two weeks.

   A trickle of dark red blood was noted from the wound during the surgery, but no bleeding was observed by the end of the case. On the first post-operative day there was a 25% hyphema, almost black in color. Intraocular pressure was 22 mm/Hg. The cornea was clear. Acetazolamide 250 mg QID and timolol maleate 0.5% BID were given along with gentamicin and prednisolone acetate 1% drops QID. The blood cleared in three weeks and the final visual acuity was 20/25.

3. A 78 year old woman was admitted on August 25, 1987 for extra-capsular cataract extraction with intraocular lens implantation. Her medical history was significant for emphysema and thyroidism. In addition she had a mild cerebrovascular accident (CVA) in March, 1987 for which she was subsequently maintained on warfarin sodium (Coumadin). Her other medications were levothyroxine sodium (Synthroid), albuterol sulfate (Proventil), and pentoxifylline (Trental).

Her neurologist discontinued her warfarin sodium five days prior to surgery. In the hospital the evening before surgery, her voice slurred and she began to perseverate. Her neurologist diagnosed a recurrence of her right hemisphere CVA and she was transferred to the Neurology Service.

A CT scan and MRI confirmed right parietal lobe hyperdensity. Heparin and then Coumadin were begun and the symptoms cleared after five days.

Methods

The study included twenty-five eyes of 22 patients undergoing planned extracapsular cataract extraction with posterior chamber intraocular lens implantation whose medical history predisposed to a bleeding disorder. Table 14-1 lists these medical indications.

Preoperatively and on the day of surgery, all patients were instructed to administer their medication as per their usual routine. Patients on aspirin received pre-operative bleeding time measurements and were included in the study if the value was greater than three minutes above normal. Patients on anticoagulants had pre-operative measurement of prothombin time (PT) and activated partial thromboplastin time (aPTT) pre-operatively and were included in the study if either was abnormal. All surgery was performed on an inpatient basis to minimize the potential for delayed bleeding.

All patients except the patient with factor XII deficiency had our routine local anesthesia consisting of intravenous midazolam (1-3 ug) and alfentanil (250–500mg) followed by retrobulbar injection of xylocaine 2% and bupivocaine 0.75% with hyaluronidase. A Honan balloon was applied

TABLE 14-1

Daily aspirin	15
Warfarin sodium	8
Dipyridamole	5
Other anticoagulants	3
Factor XII deficiency	1

(Several patients had more than one indication)

to the eye for twenty minutes at a pressure of 30 mm/Hg. During the procedure alfentanil was administered intravenously by drip or pump at a rate of .1 to .2 ug/kg/min.

The patient with severe factor XII deficiency had general anesthesia as her hematologist felt that a retrobulbar hemorrhage was potentially uncontrollable.

The surgical technique was as follows:

A speculum was placed between the lids. A traction suture of 6-0 silk was placed at the inferior limbus through clear cornea and draped over the inferior blade of the speculum. Cautery was performed to the superior limbal vascular arcade. No conjunctival dissection or manipulation was performed. A diamond knife was used to create a 2/3 corneal thickness incision of 11 mm in chord length parallel to the limbus through clear cornea 1/2 mm anterior to the limbal vascular arcade. The anterior chamber was entered by a Beaver #75 blade and the anterior chamber was filled with hyaluronic acid. The corneal incision was completed with corneoscleral scissors in a single plane. No shelving of the incision was attempted to limit trauma to the corneal endothelium.

An anterior lens capsulectomy was performed and the nucleus expressed. The residual lens cortex was aspirated with manual I/A technique. A modified J loop, no holes UV filter, 10° angled prolene haptic lens was implanted in the bag by direct observation. Acetylcholine was instilled intracamerally after lens placement. The corneal incision was closed with interrupted sutures of 10-0 nylon. No peripheral iridectomy or iridotomy was performed. Topical steroids and antibiotics were instilled beneath a sterile dressing. No subconjunctival injections were given.

The patients were examined on the first post-operative day, and then at one week, one month, two months, and three months post-operative. Each examination included slit lamp exam, keratometry, refraction, corneal pachymetry and tonometry. Specular microscopy was performed at the two months examination.

A control group was generated by reviewing the records of all patients undergoing extracapsular cataract extraction with intraocular lens implantation over the past five years who had preoperative and postoperative specular microscopy. Eleven patients were identified whose medical history or list of medications suggested them to be anticoagulated. Abnormal PT and aPTT were documented in the chart for patients on anticoagulants. Unfortunately, bleeding times were not available for those patients on aspirin. The control group consisted of:

Daily aspirin	7
Warfarin	4
Dipyridamole	3
Other anticoagulants	2

Several patients had more than one indication. All the patients in the control group had a fornix based conjunctival recession and a limbal corneoscleral incision.

Results

All patients in both groups achieved 20/40 or better final visual acuity. There were no cases of persistent corneal edema, nor of intraocular pressure greater than 24 mm/Hg on the first post-operative day. There were no cases of Descemet's membrane disinsertion or of wound leak. The complications noted are listed in Table 14-2.

The one case of retrobulbar hemorrhage in the study group was noted immediately and did not increase after the Honan balloon was placed. The intraocular pressure was measured as 10 mm/Hg after 20 minutes of compression and the surgery was performed without evidence of positive posterior pressure. Surgery in the patient with a retrobulbar hemorrhage in the control group was postponed and operated two months later without reoccurrence.

Increased with the rule astigmatism was defined as greater than or equal to three diopters more than the pre-operative measurements at the two month examination.

The patients in the study group included as being aware of their sutures subjectively complained of the foreign body sensation greater than our routine patients. For the control group, the nurse's comments in the post-op notes were reviewed for complaint of suture sensation. No mention was found. Bandage contact lenses were given to the study patients usually at the one week examination and were always removed no later than the two month examination.

Suture removal was performed no sooner than the two month examination and was necessitated by suture induced astigmatism, loose sutures, or persistent foreign body sensation.

Increased corneal thickness on the first post-operative day was defined as greater than or equal to .050 mm. greater than the preoperative value. For the study group, the corneal pachymetry at 24 hours post-operative revealed an increase in corneal thickness of 0.029 mm (0.552 pre-op, 0.581 at 24 hrs.). This is similar to the 0.026 increase in corneal thickness for the control group. By the one month examination, in all patients in both groups the corneal thickness had returned to the preoperative value.

Increased endothelial cell loss was defined as greater than 15% loss of

TABLE 14-2

		Study Patients (%)		Controls (%)	
1.	Intraocular hemorrhage	0	0	7	64
2.	Retrobulbar hemorrhage	1	4	1	9
3.	Increased with the rule astigmatism	14	56	1	9
4.	Increased awareness of sutures	10	40	0	0
5.	Bandage soft contact lens for comfort	2	8	0	0
6.	Need to remove sutures	19	76	1	9
7.	Increased corneal thickness on first post-operative day	5	20	0	0
8.	Increased endothelial cell loss	7	28	0	0

central corneal endothelium compared to preoperative values. For the study group, the endothelial cell loss was 11% compared to 6% for the control group.

Discussion

Hemostasis following vascular injury, as occurs with surgery, depends on the formation of a primary platelet plug (platelet mediated) and a secondary fibrin plug (enzymatic medicated). Various systemic diseases as well as medication may inhibit these processes.

Platelets undergo three basic reactions: adherence, release and aggregation. The primary initiators of platelet adherence are the subendothelial elements, primarily collagen, that are exposed to platelets following vascular injury. Platelet adherence to collagen is mediated by factor VII, which is found either in the plasma or bound to platelets or to endothelium. Within the platelet, thromboxane A_2 is generated via prostaglandin metabolism which cause platelets to change their shape and release granular contents. Nearby platelets are recruited and the process repeated.

The release of granules also exposes a glycoprotein complex $GPII_b$ III_a which mediates aggregation, the process by which platelets interact with each other. The primary phase of hemostasis is complete as a primary platelet plug is formed.

The secondary phase of hemostasis, coagulation, is a biologic cascade of enzymes and their substrates leading to formation of a fibrin clot. All the coagulation factors except factor VIII are synthesized in the liver. A defect anywhere along this enzymatic cascade will result in the inability to form a stable hemostatic fibrin plug.

The most commonly taken medications that interfere with hemostasis are aspirin and other non-steroidal anti-inflammatory medications. Aspirin irreversibly inactivates the enzyme cyclooxygenase, preventing the generation of thromboxane A_2. Platelets become dysfunctional for their life as they can no longer undergo release. No primary plug formation is possible.

All platelets in the circulation are affected, and normal coagulation is not possible until new platelets have replaced the existing circulation, usually requiring seven to ten days. Non-steroidal anti-inflammatory drugs other than aspirin cause a similar defect in cyclooxygenase activity, however the effect is reversible and lasts only as long as the drug is present in the circulation.

Dipyridamole (Persantine) and Sulfinpyrazone (Anturane) are two other medication often prescribed to inhibit platelet function. Their effect on hemostasis is less pronounced.

Other medication which may interfere with platelet function are: antibiotics (penicillin and derivatives), antihistamines and antitussives, calcium channel-blocking agents, diuretics, serotonin antagonists, sympathetic blocking agents, tranquilizers and antipsychotic agents, vasodilators, and xanthine derivatives.

Impairment of platelet function can be assessed by measurement of the bleeding time. Prolonged bleeding time is a non-specific indicator of a platelet disorder but signals the risk of bleeding during surgery.

Heparin and warfarin (Coumadin) are amongst the drugs that inhibit the enzymatic cascade of coagulation. These anticoagulants prevent the formation of the secondary fibrin plug.

The mode of action of heparin is mediated by antithrombin III which neutralizes thrombin and activated factors IX, X, XI, XII. In the presence of heparin, this interaction is enhanced. The duration of action is four to six hours.

Warfarin interferes with the production of vitamin K dependent coagulation factors, primarily II, VII, IX, and X. The half life of warfarin averages 36 hours, so three to five days are necessary to restore normal coagulation.

The coagulation phase of hemostasis is commonly measured by the prothrombin time (PT) and activated partial thromboplastin time (aPTT). Prolongation of the PT is seen in warfarin therapy while heparin has its greatest effect on the aPTT.[12]

Thus in taking a pre-operative history attention to these conditions is necessary with particular emphasis on drug intake. A simple negative response to an inquiry on aspirin is insufficient as many patients are unaware of the aspirin content in many over-the-counter medications. It is helpful to name several common preparations that include aspirin in order to elicit relevant medication history.

This study was undertaken to determine if cataract surgery could be safely and effectively performed in anticoagulated patients without altering their systemic medication regimen. If so, we could be more confident that surgery would not have any adverse effect on the patient's medical health.

The study design suffered from the use of retrospective controls rather than randomly assigning patients to two groups, one that received the corneal incision and the other that received the posterior limbal incision. The decision to treat all patients with corneal incision was made as our experience with the posterior limbal incision had produced intraoperative or postoperative hemorrhage often enough to discontinue this technique for the safety of our patients.

The anterior incision produced more awareness of the sutures, more with the rule astigmatism requiring suture removal, and more transient corneal edema. However, none of these factors persisted past two months and the final visual outcome was unaffected by the technique.

None of the patients had pre-operative corneal endothelial pathology. The increased trauma to the corneal endothelium from this incision may be a cause for caution in cases of pre-existing guttata or low endothelial cell density.

Several investigators have reported a lower incidence of hemorrhage after a peribulbar injection rather than a retrobulbar injection.[13-16] In this prospective study we chose to use our routine retrobulbar injection to determine if there would be a higher incidence of retrobulbar hemorrhage in these patients than in our routine population. The one retrobulbar hemorrhage in 25 study patients and one in eleven controls is inconclusive.

The safety of this technique and the absence of long term complication make this technique recommendable as an alternative to temporarily discontinuing anticoagulants.

Most important, no patient had any change in their medical health during the surgical period.

Acknowledgement

Joseph Rugierio, MD, Assistant Professor of Medicine, Cornell University Medical College, provided hematologic consultation on many of the patients in this study, reviewed the manuscript, and provided suggestions.

References

1. Kulvin, SM., IOL's and Anticoagulant therapy. American Intraocular Implant Society Journal, Vol 5, p. 37, 1979.
2. Schwartz, SR., ed. Principles of Surgery, 47th ed., New York, McGraw-Hill, Inc., p. 120, 1983.
3. Jaffe, NS., Cataract Surgery and Its Complications, 3rd ed., St. Louis, CV Mosby, p. 413, 1983.
4. Ling, R., Anticoagulants and Cataract Surgery, Ophthalmic Surgery, Vol 19(7) pp. 528–529, 1988.
5. Maida, JW., American Intraocular Implant Society Journal, Vol 5, p. 36, 1979.
6. Hall, DL., American Intraocular Implant Society Journal, Vol 5, p. 37, 1979.
7. Hall, DL., Steen, WH., Drummond, JW., Anticoagulants and Cataract Surgery. Annals of Ophthalmology, Vol 12, pp. 759–60, 1980.
8. Hall, DL., Steen, WH., Drummond, JW., Byrd, WA., Anticoagulants and Cataract Surgery, Ophthalmic Surgery, Vol 19(3), pp. 221–2, 1988.
9. McMahon, LB., Anticoagulants and Cataract Surgery. Journal Cataract and Refractive Surgery. Vol 14, p. 569, 1988.
10. Gainey, SP., Robertson, DM., Ray W., Ilstrup, D., Ocular Surgery on Patients Receiving Long-term Warfarin Therapy. American Journal of Ophthalmology. Vol 108, pp. 142–146, 1989.
11. Stone, LS., Kline, OR., Sklar, C., Intraocular Lenses and Anticoagulation and Antiplatelet Therapy. American Intraocular Implant Society Journal, Vol 11, pp. 165–8, 1985.
12. Ansell, JE. Handbook of Hemostasis and Thrombosis, Boston. Little Brown and Company, 1986.
13. Gills, JP, Anesthesia for Cataract Extraction (letter) Ophthalmic Surgery, 17: 173, 1986.
14. Davis, DB II, Mandel Mr: Posterior Peribulbar Anesthesia. An Alternative to Retrobulbar Anesthesia. Journal Cataract Refractive Surgery. 12:182–184, 1986.

15. Bloomer, LB, Administration of Periocular Anesthesia. Journal Cataract Refractive Surgery 12:677–679, 1986.
16. Wang, HS, Peribulbar Anesthesia for Ophthalmic Procedures. Journal Cataract Refractive Surgery, 14:441–443, 1988.

Chapter 15

ROUNDTABLE DISCUSSION HIGH RISK PATIENTS AND SURGICAL COMPLICATIONS

Calvin W. Roberts, MD, Moderator

Roberts: For this Round Table, what I have in mind is to talk a little bit about the thoughts that cataract surgeons should have in terms of the corneal endothelium. Obviously, what we're trying to avoid—cases of bullous keratopathy—was commonly seen in patients with iris-fixated intraocular lenses. Since that time, we have all grown to appreciate the importance of the corneal endothelium. In evaluating corneal endo- thelium, we start at the slit lamp looking for evidence of epithelial edema and stromal edema, and looking for the presence of folds in Descemet's membrane—which are indicative of corneal edema—and we use our slit lamp to try to get a specular reflection (Figure 15-1). I think this is a technique all of you do routinely, and you know how to angle your slit lamp beam at high magnification to get a very good and clear view of the corneal endothelium. It's something I really encourage you to do routinely. Other techniques for evaluating the endothelium start with the pachymeter which is a physiologic means of assessing the endothelium. There are different types of pachyme- ters—the light pachymeter that fits on the Haag-Streit slit lamp, ultra- sonic pachymeters, and the pachymeter we built into the specular microscope. When it comes to specular microscopy, the area has really grown in the last 10 years. It was actually just 10 years ago, in 1980, that Dr. Charles Koester and I actually put out the first of the wide field specular microscopes. When it comes to evaluating patients with the specular microscope, obviously the first concern is cell density. This picture that comes from Herb Kaufman and Bill Bourne's original papers using the conventional small field specular microscope shows how normal patients will have a decrease in cell count from childhood to old age (Figure 15-2). More recently, as we've gotten more sophis- ticated with the specular microscope, we're concerned about cell mor- phology—things called polymegathism and polymorphism. Polyme- gathism refers to difference in size of cells in the field. Polymorphism has to do with difference in shapes.

This is a case of a patient with a lot of polymegathism (Figure 15-3). You see there are small cells and big cells in the same field. This is a

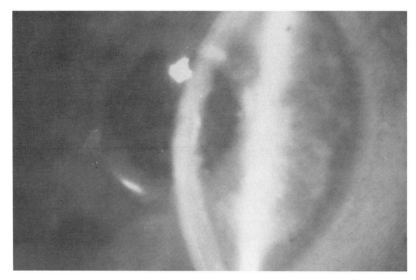

Figure 15-1:   Use of a slit lamp to look for epithelial edema and stromal edema, and looking for the presence of folds in Descemet's membrane.

patient with polymorphism (Figure 15-4). You see there are a lot of cells that are irregular; there are cells that appear round; there are cells that appear stretched; there are cells that have five sides; there are cells with six sides, and there are cells with seven sides. The question often asked

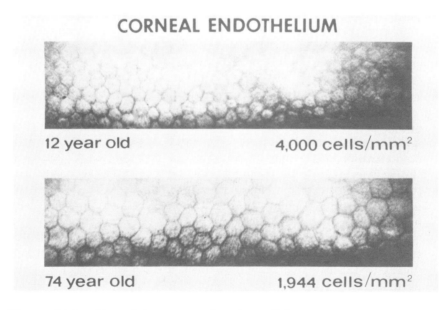

Figure 15-2:   Use of the conventional small field specular microscope to show how normal patients will have a decrease in cell count from childhood to old age.

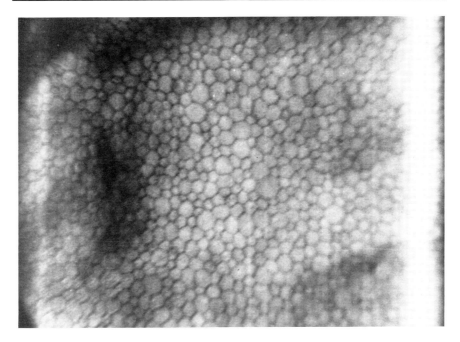

Figure 15-3:   A case of a patient with a lot of polymegathism.

is, "which are the patients that should be receiving specular microscopy?" Certainly, this is not a technique that you would routinely want to use on all your patients. I think of these as my criteria for having a patient undergo specular microscopy: 1) a patient who has problems with the other eye, 2) a patient who's had previous surgery—and several studies have shown that long-standing glaucoma will have an adverse effect on the corneal endothelium, and 3) a patient who is having a secondary IOL. I use a specular microscopy to assess how much trauma occurred to the endothelium in the primary operation, and to determine how much reserve there is left in the cornea. Certainly, I do this for patients with endothelial dystrophy.

Now, what I would like to do with the Round Table, is ask not so much what the panelists would do with various patients, but actually to find out what are their thought processes. I think we can learn a lot from thinking or hearing about what other people think about in various types of patients. So, I present this as our first patient for the Round Table. This is a 72 year old man with a 20 year history of primary open angle glaucoma (Figure 15-5). He has had an argon laser trabeculoplasty, and has also had a trabeculectomy. He now has a cataract. His ocular medications are pilocarpine and Timoptic. Now, I throw this out at Hal. I'm going to put you on the spot first to say that these are patients that we see often. What do you think about in terms of the cornea in a patient like this? Let's, for a second, think not of their glaucoma problem, but is there anything special that you would be looking for in terms of the cornea?

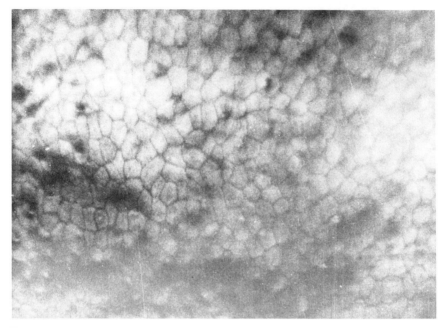

Figure 15-4: A case of a patient with polymorphism.

Balyeat: Tell me this, is the trabeculectomy functioning?

Roberts: Yes, it's a functioning trabeculectomy.

Balyeat: Well, I mean the patient still is maintained on pilocarpine and Timoptic, so it can't be . . .

Roberts: Partially . . .

Balyeat: I think because of his previous surgical history and also because of his prolonged history of chronic open angle glaucoma, assuming that his cornea looked all right during a routine slit lamp examination, I probably would do a pachymetry measurement on him but probably not specular microscopy without any other indications of potential corneal decompensation.

Roberts: So that in your experience a patient like this would be pretty safe for cataract surgery assuming that their corneal thickness was normal. John?

Hunkeler: I wouldn't assume anything. First off, you really haven't given us much of a history. We don't know anything about the patient's visual field status, and that would change my thinking considerably as to whether or not the pressure was controlled adequately. That's the determination I'm a little concerned about—the patients on pilocarpine and Timoptic. Whatever I end up doing will be very seriously determined by what the heck is going on in the other eye. You haven't told us anything about that. This is, the way it's presented, a one-eyed patient. I would approach this with an extreme level of caution, unless I know exactly what is going on with the other eye. I assume it's no light perception. I will approach this a very conservative way. But a lot of it would be determined by what the visual field status is and evaluating the cornea becomes somewhat of a technical problem.

Roberts: If we look at this as a normal endothelium for someone who is 72 years old—the normal cell count would be approximately 2500— this patient has a cell count of approximately 1600. So, now I throw it back to you, John. This is the only eye of this patient with a cell count of 1600. Is there any way, assuming that we assess the cataract surgery is necessary, to try to restore some vision? Is the fact that the patient has a 1600 cell count in any way going to affect your technique?

Hunkeler: Yes, it probably will. I will be depending on the size of the pupil, the density of the nucleus, and be more inclined to do a planned extracapsular procedure, because I'm aware of the increased amount of manipulation in my hands that would be required to emulsify the nucleus. I would be more inclined to do a planned extracapsular procedure, and with the presence of the previous filtration, probably do a clear corneal incision. If I assess that the intraocular pressure is inadequately controlled, I would probably do a separate trabeculectomy at the same time at a new site.

Roberts: David?

Apple: Maybe I can make a few general comments. Certainly, financial considerations aside, I think viscoelastic is immensely important. One might worry about a glaucoma patient using viscoelastic because, as you said earlier, the post-op pressure rises, but we've just recently done some experiments with video showing that if you just get in there and take out the Healon—Healon comes out very quickly—we were pleasantly surprised. So, perhaps post-op pressure rise is one major excuse for not using Healon or something like it. I would be sure to get it all out, to protect the cornea. In terms of the glaucoma, we've done some experiments looking at these cadaver eyes from the side. People talk about how glaucoma can actually get better after posterior chamber lens implantation. I think that the reason is extremely simple. The crystalline lens is like 4mm thick; an IOL is like 0.3mm thick. When you look sideways at these eyes, and we've done lots of this now, you've just collapsed everything into kind of a membrane; you've got a little bigger . . . and opened up anterior chamber after a posterior chamber lens. So, maybe that can actually assist in improving glaucoma. Would you like to comment on that?

Roberts: It's interesting. If you look at the size of the anterior chamber after cataract surgery, as opposed to before, and if you go on the basis that the anterior chamber has a volume of approximately 0.250ml and

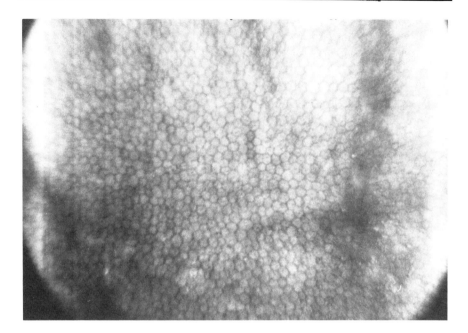

Figure 15-5: View of a 72 year old man with a 20 year history of primary open angle glaucoma.

the posterior chamber has a volume of approximately 0.060ml, the lens has a volume of approximately 0.250ml. So, the posterior chamber lens has a volume actually of about 0.035ml. If you add this all up and take out the lens and put in a posterior chamber lens, you effectively double the size of your anterior chamber. This is going to have an impact upon the fluid dynamics that are occurring in the angle.

Apple: That's right. Looking at pictures that I've done but don't have here, it's striking. It's amazing. I think people have underemphasized this fact. So, I think the idea of glaucoma that's improved with IOL is a real one. I think certainly capsular fixation to minimize the scraping is also important in the whole pattern.

Roberts: This second patient is a 75 year old woman who underwent intracapsular cataract extraction 12 years ago (Figure 15-6). She has been wearing an extended wear soft contact lens. Over the past year, she has had episodes of a red, painful eye with blurred vision. She asks whether she would be a candidate for a secondary intraocular lens. My question to you is, what thoughts would go into your mind as you were examining this patient?

Balyeat: Assuming that the other eye is a normal eye, I think this patient is a good candidate for consideration of a secondary lens implant. There are two or three factors. One, the fact that she is wearing an extended wear contact lens increases her risk of corneal disease through infec-

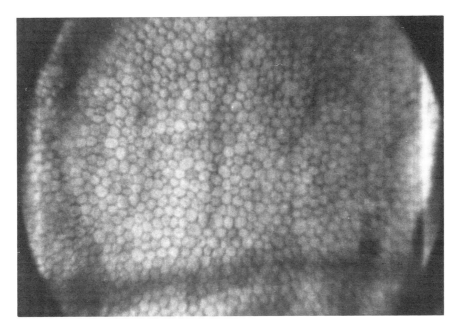

Figure 15-6: View of a 75-year-old woman who underwent intracapsular extraction 12 years ago.

tion, primarily. This may also represent the fact that she is unable to insert and remove daily wear contact lenses on her own. The complication rate with secondary lens implantation, I think, is acceptable although it certainly is higher than the complication rate after primary procedures. Another consideration is whether or not she has vitreous in her anterior chamber. Although it always should be a consideration, I'm not impressed that the complication rate of secondary lens implantation with vitreous in the anterior chamber is any greater than if there is no vitreous in the anterior chamber. So, again, assuming the cornea is in good shape, through either pachymetry or specular microscopy, then I would say she would be an excellent candidate. I would further say that this would be a patient that I would use an anterior chamber lens, as opposed to a transclerally-fixed posterior chamber lens.

Roberts: John?

Hunkeler: Basically, I agree with what Hal just said. I think a lot of my planning and thinking about this particular case—what the patient would have to do with the appearance of the iris and any peripheral anterior synechiae—that it may be impossible actually to put an anterior chamber lens in this patient with an intracapsular surgery, where there are roughly four to six clock hours of anterior synechiae. So, with that in mind, I would have to consider whether or not an epikeratophakia might be a better choice than a sclerally-fixated lens. I would also incorporate in my thinking, besides the appearance of the cornea, any history of cystoid macular edema in the past—getting a good look at the peripheral retina and, among other things, making sure there is not any pre-existing retinal surgery. Those things would mitigate against intraocular surgery and be pro-epikeratophakia.

Roberts: What concerned me about this patient was not that she had episodes of red eye, but that they were associated with blurred vision. Blurred vision made me think maybe she was getting corneal edema from the contact lenses. It turned out that this lady had a cell count of just around 1000 cells/mm2. Usually we think about 700 as the minimum cut-off for maintaining corneal clarity, so that in a hypoxic state potentially her corneal endothelium could not function properly and that is why she was getting corneal edema. A question again for the panelists—do you have cut-offs in terms of cell counts for patients for secondary IOLs? Would the fact that this lady had a cell count of 1000 encourage you or discourage you from doing secondary IOLs, and encourage you or discourage you from doing an epi?

Hunkeler: Given a cell count of 1000—let's work around that—if I am going to have to do a lot of intraocular manipulation with either a sclerally-fixated lens or a lot of anterior segment iris reconstruction, I'd be reluctant to do a lot of those manipulations with that cell count and would consider the alternative—an epikeratophakia. Her age is getting a little advanced and could pose difficulties with wound healing and dry eyes with epikeratophakia. But, if she had adequate tear function she should do well with an epi. I would be more inclined to do an epi than having to do more intraocular manipulation.

Balyeat: I would be inclined to do a secondary lens implant with that cell count using viscoelastic, assuming that her iris and angle were in relatively good health. So, again, you wouldn't have to manipulate the anterior segment too much. But, I would use probably a pachymetry measurement again as one of my determinants, and if the pachymetry measurement was over about 0.6mm, I would certainly be less inclined— and this is after she's had her contact lens out for a while—I'd be less inclined to jump in and do anything.

Roberts: David?

Apple: So many people are telling us to never use anterior chamber lenses again. I think we really have to be careful in discussing this. I think that it's really worth repeating that the open-looped, flexible anterior chamber lenses we have now are a world apart from the old, closed-loop lenses that give anterior chamber lenses a bad name. Say that I were totally healthy except for just needing a secondary implant. I think the decision might be determined by my location. If you are at a corneal center with a physician who does dozens of the sutured lenses, that's fine. But out in the real world I think you are much better off, all things being equal, with a relatively healthy eye with no glaucoma, to go with the Kelman modification, open-looped type anterior chamber lenses. They're so much simpler.

Roberts: For me, what the cell count does is change my thinking in terms of whether to put in a posterior chamber lens or an anterior chamber lens. In my hands, trying to sew in a posterior chamber lens in someone without a posterior capsule, involves a lot more trauma to the anterior segment and potentially greater cell loss. So, in a patient like this with a cell count of 1000, I would be much more likely to put in an anterior chamber lens if I felt it could be done relatively atraumatically than to try to go sew in a posterior chamber lens.

Finally, I want to talk about patients with endothelial dystrophy. The question comes up—when do you do a combined procedure; that is, a triple procedure including a corneal transplant along with our cataract extraction? How important with patients with endothelial dystrophy is pachymetry versus the actual cell count?

This next patient is a 66 year old woman who had a triple procedure— a penetrating keratoplasty with extracapsular cataract extraction and a posterior chamber IOL for cataract and Fuchs' dystrophy (Figure 15-7). She realized that it took her close to a year until she got her best possible acuity and she has 4.5D of corneal astigmatism from her corneal transplant. She asked whether it would be possible to remove the cataract that she now has in her other eye without doing a corneal transplant. John?

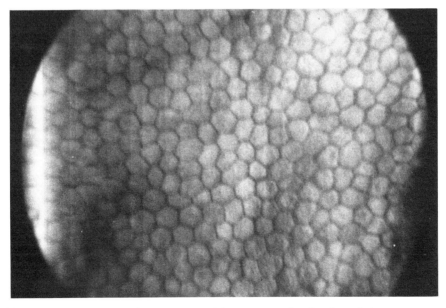

Figure 15-7:   View of a 66-year-old woman who had a triple procedure.

Hunkeler: I've heard all sorts of different surgeons try to get around this problem. The most recent was a patient on whom I had recommended a combined penetrating keratoplasty, cataract extraction and lens implantation. She went to another physician who said, "Yes, you have corneal edema and a cataract in that eye, but we can fix up the other eye quicker. We'll just do the cataract extraction and put in a lens implant." You can guess what happened. She ended up with corneal edema in both eyes. It doesn't make a whole lot of sense as to why he did that. Anyway, that being the case, you'd have to assess this second eye very carefully—whether the corneal thickness was over 0.6mm, and looking at the endothelial cell count. That would help me to determine whether or not to attempt to do the procedure without a keratoplasty. If it's a borderline situation with no corneal edema, no history of morning edema, I'd be inclined to do it. I've gotten away with doing it. If necessary, you can always come back at a later date and add in the keratoplasty as a separate procedure. It may add a couple of months of morbidity for the patient, but certainly that is an option.

Roberts: Do you have guidelines, John? Do you have guidelines about corneal thickness?

Hunkeler: If it's over 0.6mm I will compare that with the other eye. I think trying to measure an absolute number is near impossible. Depending on the cell count and the pachymetry—0.61mm or 0.62mm— I am more inclined to hold off. When both numbers get off a higher pachymetry of 0.63mm and a cell count of 600 or so, then that inclines me more and more towards the keratoplasty.

Roberts: Hal?

Balyeat: Since I don't do keratoplasty, I generally feel that using 0.6mm as a cut-off is a fairly reasonable way to go. I agree with John. Generally what I'll do is if a patient has confluent guttatae, but relatively thin corneas—then I will suggest to them that they have a cataract extraction and lens implant. But, I certainly think that the patient deserves a significant amount of counseling both in this situation and also the situation when their corneal thickness is increased. I spend a great deal of time telling them that the morbidity is going to be higher, etc., but I certainly feel that it is in their best interests to have a combined procedure rather than undergo a cataract extraction and subsequently end up having to have keratoplasty.

Balyeat: David, you have a comment?

Apple: I agree pretty much.

Roberts: I think the point to remember in patients with Fuchs dystrophy is that the guttatae are greater centrally, and that they are less dense in the periphery. So, patients with Fuchs dystrophy will tend to get their corneal edema earlier centrally, and it will progress peripherally. Dr. Balyeat talked about the confluent guttatae. The presence of gut-tatae does not correlate with the endothelial cell count. I will show you two patients whose slit lamp examinations look similar in terms of their extensive guttatae, but the cell counts are very different. These pictures are all the same magnification. This patient's cells—that you can see in between the guttatae—are small (Figure 15-8). Here the cells are much larger, comparing these cells to those cells (Figure 15-9). Now, the patient with the smaller cells and the higher cell count would be much more likely to do well after having the cataract oper-ation, than the patient with the larger endothelial cells and the greater amount of dystrophy. So, I think the message here is that the slit lamp exam that just shows the presence of guttatae should not be the end-all in terms of evaluating these patients. Most important in my hands in evaluating these patients, is the corneal thickness. This agrees with the other speakers. I am maybe a little bit more liberal in terms of corneal thickness with which I'll do just a cataract extraction. I usually use a cut-off of approximately 0.65mm in corneal thickness as my cut-off for when to do a triple procedure and when to just do the cataract. The specular microscopy is hard in these patients because you often can't see the endothelium because of all the guttatae. But this is an area that is always interesting for me—when a patient comes in with corneal dystrophy and cataract, and I have to try to figure it out,

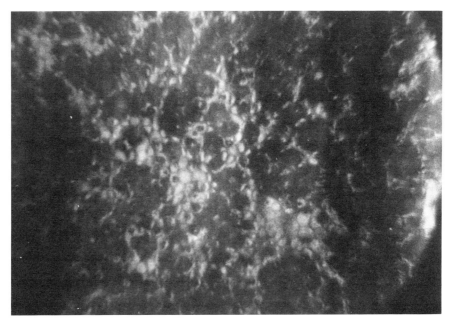

Figure 15-8:   View of a patient's cells in between the guttatae that are small.

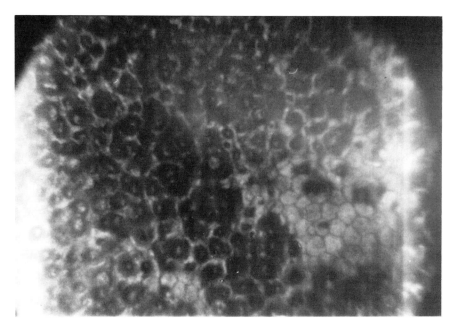

Figure 15-9:   View of a patient's cells that are much larger.

counsel them, and think about the benefits of the faster rehabilitation without the corneal graft, and the risks of corneal edema if we don't do the graft. Does anyone have anything to add? No? Thank you.

Chapter 16

ROUNDTABLE DISCUSSION POTPOURRI: COMPARING SURGICAL CLOSURE TECHNIQUES & MANAGEMENT OF THE CATARACT PATIENT

C. William Simcoe, MD, Moderator

Many surgeons are contemplating whether they should proceed with extracapsular cataract extraction or convert to phacoemulsification. I would like to present some "food for thought" on both procedures and in defense of the manual technique of extracapsular surgery.

One must remember that most of the surgeons in the United States and the rest of the world still use the extracapsular technique of cataract extraction. Some surgeons do not have the luxury of automated phacoemulsification units as cost containment in their areas may be restrictive. Some surgeons prefer the control exhibited by the manual technique over automated systems. Whatever the reason, surgical results in these areas are identical to those using automated systems as long as the surgeon is proficient in his technique.

Many surgeons and hospitals in the United States are now feeling the crunch of diminishing Medicare reimbursements and cost containment. Expenditures for the purchasing of IOLs and equipment are being limited. Foldable IOLs and phacoemulsification may yield as good a visual acuity result as extracapsular surgery, but at what cost to the patient and the Medicare/third party system?

I prefer extracapsular cataract extraction. In fact, I still use the traditional "can opener" capsulotomy via small radial punctures within the anterior capsule, making sure that my 30-gauge sharp needle cystotome with irrigation does not engage the nucleus. The irrigation from the cystotome is used to create hydrodissection of the nucleus.

Nucleus delivery is accomplished with a Simcoe lens loop. This instrument has an anterior serrated side to cradle and grasp the nucleus. The curved tip is maneuvered from the vertical to horizontal position within the eye to retract the iris and, once within the bag, to deliver the nucleus without creating vitreal pressure as in traditional nucleus delivery.

Once the wound is closed, following nucleus delivery with temporary sutures, I use the Simcoe irrigation and aspiration apparatus, a twin cannula unit with fluid injected either by gravity or by a hand-held bulb. Aspiration is via a syringe connected to the cannula via tubing. The twin cannula system has a very thin profile and allows less wound leakage during I&A than automated systems.

Once I&A begins, cortex must be engaged blindly within the periphery of the capsular bag, hidden by the overlying iris. The Simcoe cannula allows this maneuver to occur in relative safety since the cannula is curved with its aspiration port facing anteriorly. If the cannula is placed deeply within the bag, cortex may be engaged without incorporating the anterior capsule and tearing zonules in the process. Since the eye is a closed chambered system due to the temporary sutures, the capsular bag remains open, making I&A easier and lessening the chances of expulsive hemorrhage.

Cortex should be engaged in the peripheral capsular bag and then stripped toward the center of the pupil where it can be aspirated under direct visualization. Once the aspiration port is occluded with cortex, the aspiration pressure proximal to the obstruction skyrockets until the cortex is cleared and the port is once again open. At this point there is a surge of built up aspiration pressure that can result in momentary shallowing of the chamber. If the cannula is held still within the eye and the aspiration port is pointing upward, there is no risk of incorporating and tearing the posterior capsule. I&A of 12 o'clock cortex is easier in extracapsular surgery since the size of the wound is larger and the gentle curve of the Simcoe cannula allows for easy access and aspiration of cortex in areas that a phacoemulsification unit would have difficulty in accomplishing.

I have always been a believer of C looped IOLs. As confirmed by Dr. David Apple's chapter, C looped IOLs distribute the fixation pressure within the capsular bag, decreasing the risk of posterior capsular striae and extrusion of the IOL from the capsular bag postoperatively. Many surgeons dislike the long haptic C loops due to the difficulty of their implantation. I disagree. Implantation of full C looped IOLs can be accomplished with ease following either capsulotomy or capsulorhexis. The key to implantation of C looped IOLs is the placement of that section of the inferior haptic proximal to the optic within the capsular bag first, allowing the remainder of the haptic to follow. The superior haptic can be either dialed into the bag or placed within the bag by forceps under direct visualization.

Following IOL placement, I perform a small peripheral iridotomy to prevent postoperative pseudophakic pupillary block glaucoma. The wound is closed with figure of eight sutures.

In summary, the manual technique of extracapsular cataract extraction with posterior chamber lens implantation is a time proven procedure which yields excellent results with minimal expenditure and should remain as the mainstay of cataract surgery.

With that editorial comment being made, I would like to now ask the panel about their cataract closures as well as pre and postoperative care of their patients.

Simcoe: I would like to ask the panel about their cataract closures as well as their pre- and postoperative care of patients.

Roberts: One of the areas I would like to comment on is the use of absorbable versus non-absorbable sutures in closing cataract wounds. I've always used 10-0 nylon and I'm really concerned about the decay of my wound over time. In particular, there are some wounds that decay a lot and some that don't decay at all. If all wounds are closed the same, why is that? Someone suggested that I do a retrospective study and look at the preoperative astigmatism. It seems that those patients who start out preoperatively with "against the rule" astigmatism tend to decay more than those patients who start out with "with the rule" astigmatism. I have no data to support that. Norman Buys from Sunnyvale, California was the first to talk to me about the use of nonabsorbable sutures. He did a prospective study looking at 10-0 nylon versus 10-0 polyester sutures. He had rather dramatic data showing much less decay in astigmatism with nonabsorbable sutures than with absorbable sutures. Do you have any experience with nonabsorbable sutures?

Simcoe: A brief summary of my experience with sutures starts way back before we even used nylon. We used 7-0 silk in residency, then 8-0 silk came along and we thought that was so wonderful that there would never be anything better. Of course, those eyes were hot and inflamed, with necrosis of tissue around the silk, which we removed three weeks later, resulted in very little astigmatism. Then, we went to nylon. Those eyes were so quiet and so lovely but I got some high cylinders because I tended to tie them too tight. Later, I found that they too would dissolve and so I went to prolene. I've used prolene for a number of years and like it very much. It doesn't dissolve, at least significantly, for a long, long time. I tried mersilene for a while but I found I had a little more cylinder that lasted longer. I know Hal has experience. Hal, tell us about it.

Balyeat: I use 10-0 mersilene. I'm not sure I use it for the right reasons. I used to use nylon and I developed a cluster of patients who had a toxicity to the nylon three years ago. They developed some rather significant inflammatory responses. As a result, I switched. I used prolene in the early 80's, but had difficulty originally because a couple of knots came loose. I think it was because I tied them incorrectly. So, I went back to prolene and subsequently the mersilene. I might add that the suture toxicity that you see with nylon also can be seen with mersilene and prolene, so it is certainly not unique to the nylon suture. The main reason that I prefer prolene or mersilene is due to the degradation of the nylon product. Seeing patients two and three years down the line after surgery, coming in with foreign body sensation and having those sutures that you have to remove, that became enough of a problem that I thought it worth the transition. Prolene and mersilene are both a little more difficult to deal with. I use a running suture and I'm convinced that one of the problems with astigmatism in planned extracapsular surgery is the fact that most of us creep up onto the surgical limbus a little too far. Sometimes that occurs as a result of our previous experience with a hyphema the last time we operated. If you are willing to put up with a slight increase in the hyphema rate, which will occur if your incision is far enough posterior, then you can remarkably reduce the incidence of high astigmatism. I'm like Bill; if I had my choice I'd leave all my patients $-1.00 + 2.00 \times 90°$. The problem with that is although mersilene reduces the drift, it doesn't eliminate it. So, many of those patients eventually end up with the cylinder axis somewhere around 165 or 180 degrees. Fortunately, the amount of cylinder diminishes also.

Simcoe: Some years ago, Dr. Henry Gelender of Dallas reported on a series of cases (AJO 1982;94:528-33) referred to him, where when sutures were later removed at the slit lamp, they developed some infections. They had some endophthalmitis; they had wound dehiscences. I wondered how that could be from suture removal. Yet, it never happened to me until about two years ago. Then, lightning struck. I operated on my receptionist's grandmother's cataract. She lived in a neighboring state. She did fine; she came back at a later time with some cylinder, so I took out a stitch. She then developed an endophthalmitis. How many of you know of cases of hypopyon following removal of a suture? Sure, it does occur. So, I changed my regimen. When they come into my office now I put in some antibiotic solution—neomycin/polymyxin/bacitracin, whatever you want to use—and then I put in a Betadine solution at half strength. A report two or three years ago showed how Betadine combined with topical antibiotics would give cultures that were 97% or 98% sterile. I also give them some Keflex 500mg to take home. I have them take that twice a day for about three days.

Let's go on and I'll ask the panelists what their pre- and postop regimes and medications are and why. Cal?

Roberts: One of the things that differentiates my care is that I give everybody indomethacin by mouth preoperatively. The dose is relative to weight. Small people get 50mg the morning of surgery; large people get 75mg. The reason is for CME purposes, and somewhat less for postoperative inflammation. Topical drops don't seem to have a lot of effect on CME. By giving the indomethacin right before the surgery, it seems to have a reasonable anti-inflammatory effect without having much of an anti-coagulant effect.

Simcoe: Since their stomachs are empty, do they get gastric irritation from just that single, small dose?

Roberts: That has not been a problem. There are some people who need to take a little antacid with it. We give preoperative topical antibiotics for three days. We give them a bottle of gentamycin to use four times a day before surgery. We use 2% cyclogel and 2.5% phenylephrine. We don't use Ocufen; using that in conjunction with systemic indomethacin is overkill. Postoperatively I don't give any injections; I give only topical drops, gentamycin drops and prednisolone acetate drops.

Balyeat: I don't treat the patients preoperatively with any systemic or topical medications, antibiotics in particular. The patients are dilated with a combination of phenylephrine and homatropine. I do use subconjunctival injections, antibiotics and Celestone, ½ cc of each. One thing I have done over the last few years is give the medication prior to the procedure as opposed to following the procedure. Again, perhaps for the wrong reason. The main reason I began before was that that was the one thing that patients would complain of at the completion of the procedure. Oftentimes, the effects of the anesthetic had worn off. I would inject them and they'd start complaining of a burning sensation. They will tell you that is the one thing about the procedure they found objectionable. If you believe in prophylactic antibiotics, it makes sense to have the antibiotics on board prior to the incision, as opposed to following the completion of the procedure. There are some downsides. You sometimes get some conjunctival chemosis inferiorly, and sometimes it's enough that it might possibly interfere with the procedure. If that starts to happen, you can discontinue the medication and use the rest of it at the end of the procedure. Occasionally you get a little bleeding inferiorly, but it is a system that works and the patients then don't have the complaints of pain. Postoperatively, I treat them with topical antibiotics, usually in the form of polypred or something of that nature. I tried Pred-G; it seemed to make sense as I was using Gentamycin to continue with that, but the patients had a significant amount of corneal toxicity with the medication. So, if you use Gentamycin, it's probably better to use it alone, and then as Cal does, with an additional anti-inflammatory. I do that for about three weeks, and then have them switch over to FML and use that for an extended period—usually about six months total.

Simcoe: At surgery I put an antibiotic drop into the cul-de-sac along with some half-strength Betadine. I do use preop topical antibiotics prophylactically and my patients take antibiotics orally after surgery. I may be treating the doctor, but there are some basic reasons. Some years ago I was a guest at the Minnesota Academy Meeting, and Dr. Lindstrom's retina-vitreous staff presented several cases of people with low grade vitritis from six months or more after surgery. They did vitreous taps, and in every single case cultured out S. epidermidis (S. albus). These were all cases of low grade, smoldering infection by an organism not virulent enough to overwhelm the eye. They would treat it with recurrent grades of treatment, but the darned stuff was back there and just hung on. I used to see some hypopyons after surgery, in the early days of cataract extraction and lens implantation, but I also had seen them in the days before lens implantation. So, when everybody said, "Well, those are 'hot lot' intraocular lenses or have polishing compound left on them," I wasn't so sure. When you see a patient the day after surgery, there are flare and cells in the anterior chamber along with protein and white blood cells, which means there is no blood aqueous barrier at that time and for a few days. So, whatever antibiotic you have a blood level of, will get in the surgically inflamed eye. I started using Keflex 500mg orally. Patients use it for about three days after surgery. I have not seen a single hypopyon in the five or six years since I started using it. For me, it works. It may not be scientific. We had one endophthalmitis years ago that ended up badly before I started this. So, on any intraocular procedure that I do including removing a stitch, I give Keflex 500mg twice a day for three days. I also inject subconjunctival Gentamycin and Decadron at the time of surgery.

Roberts: I would like to bring up the frequency of visits postop. I see patients at one day, one week, one month, and two months postop. I think the most important concern is to detect the patient with endophthalmitis early. There is a peak time for endophthalmitis at about five days. If you aren't going to see patients for a week's time, as I don't, it's really important in postop teaching to tell them to call in for anything that seems worrisome.

Balyeat: I pretty much do the same thing. I see them at 24 hours, then at a week, then usually six weeks at which time their glasses are dispensed. I think we owe it to the patients to fully inform them what to anticipate postoperatively. The office staff can do an invaluable service here. The thing that bothers me the most is an individual who comes in postoperatively with a retinal detachment. For instance, that individual may have called the office and was put off for a routine examination. That's a real disservice. Certainly the same thing would hold true of something more emergent, but I think the office staff really needs to be informed and to get the postoperative patients back if they have any questions at all. What patients call and complain frequently of are small hyphemas that occur postoperatively within the first week or 10 days. Many of those patients have some obscuration of vision that will last transiently, but may be fairly significant lasting for 24 hours or so. I generally see those patients, although I know that when they call they've had a painless decrease in their visual acuity. The overwhelming majority of those will have a small hyphema, usually a microscopic hyphema which will layer out. Many of the patients will not see clearly in the morning, then as the day goes on their vision gets much better because of the effect of gravity on the hyphema.

Simcoe: The important point that he makes, and I agree, is that we should tell the patient that any discomfort or any change in their vision should signal that they call us immediately. People who are developing endophthalmitis will almost always have pain. They will certainly have a decrease in vision, or they're having a detachment or a hyphema or whatever. So, we give them printed instructions to call us.

(Questions and Answers from the audience moderated by Dr. Rodney Kalil were then entertained.)

QUESTION: How long after surgery do you continue topical antibiotics in uncomplicated cases, and why? Do you continue the antibiotics as long as you continue the steroids?

Simcoe: My patients will use the 5ml topical generic polymyxin/neomycin/bacitracin and steroid drops four times a day until they are empty.

Roberts: Our patients continue the antibiotics for a week, but they continue their steroids for six weeks.

Balyeat: I use it for three weeks, and then switch over to an anti-inflammatory without any topical antibiotic.

Simcoe: By the way, if you do remove a suture to reduce astigmatism, stop the steroids a good two weeks ahead of time, or you'll get some wound dehiscence or some cylinder against the rule. Stop the steroids well in advance of when you are going to nick the suture.

QUESTION: Does any of the panel use antibiotic-saturated collagen shields at the time of surgery?

Simcoe: I have not, but I've thought about it.

Roberts: I have not, and I've not thought about it.

Balyeat: Neither have I.

QUESTION: In regard to astigmatism, does any of the panel use an operative keratometer at the time of surgery?

Simcoe: I did once, and don't now. I wasn't that successful with it. It didn't seem to help me that much.

Roberts: The operative keratometer is a really tricky instrument. The optics require several things, most important is to have a normal intraocular pressure. If your intraocular pressure is low or high, it's going to distort the mires and give you inaccurate readings. So, unless you are really in good control of the postoperative intraocular pressure at the end of the case, which I think you would be very surprised to find that you're not if you want to actually measure it, it's not all that accurate. Dick Keats did a paper about measurement of the cylinder at the time of and after surgery. He measured it later and found that there was no significant difference in terms of six-month astigmatism with patients that had operative keratometry and those that had not.

Balyeat: Some years ago, I studied three groups of patients prospectively. I looked at 50 patients prior to the use of an intraoperative keratometer; then did 50 patients with a Terry keratometer; then did an additional 50 patients without a Terry keratometer. I found out that the second group, those with the Terry keratometer reading, and the third group without the Terry keratometer reading after I'd had experience, were identical and I had less astigmatism in those two groups than I did in the group prior to the use of the intraoperative keratometer. So, I think that the keratometer is helpful. It is somewhat time-consuming, expensive and cumbersome. My routine now is to use one of the disposable or easily accessible keratometers. There are a variety of them available. When you are in the operating room, you need to start looking at these things and then predict what your postoperative cylinder is going to be. Then, when you see the patient the next day or at his 1-week visit, have your ophthalmic assistant do a refraction and perhaps keratometry measurements, and then you'll find out gradually how good you are and you'll reach an end point where you'll know pretty much what cylinder you are inducing. I would agree with Cal that the single most important thing is the degree of intraocular pressure. There are, of course, devices available to allow you to determine that. I think you can use your clinical judgment and be fairly accurate in assuming that the pressure is going to be somewhere in the range of 20mmHg.

Simcoe: I've always kept a Schiotz tonometer on the operating table. I would try, in a case when I was using the keratometer, to measure the pressure. Even doing this, astigmatism was inconsistent.

Roberts: I bought a keratometer. In my hospital I share the O.R. with an innumerable number of people. They all complained because it cut down working distance and they found they were always banging into it. So, they made me take the thing off.

QUESTION: Nylon used to be considered a permanent suture, but now it's an absorbable suture. Is there any indication for using an absorbable suture alone or in combination with non-absorbable in extracapsular surgery?

Roberts: I think it would be interesting to put a couple of inert sutures at 12 o'clock and finish the rest of your wound, if you're doing a planned extracapsular with nylon. You get a little more support to prevent delayed drift, without having to worry about having to cut sutures.

Simcoe: The trouble is, it takes nylon a long time to dissolve. It doesn't happen in three to four months or so. The guys in my area who use the nylon are forever picking little barbed wires out of the corneas of their patients. But sometimes it's a year, two, three until that happens. So, I don't know that it would dissolve soon enough to really help you.

Balyeat: I don't have any experience with absorbable sutures. I've used a running suture ever since I started doing cataract surgery. It behooves you to be careful about your wound, because as we all know, you can't cut those sutures prematurely. If you are using that totally non-absorbable suture, you do have to cut one—for instance a prolene or a mersilene—those have a tendency to be very uncomfortable for the patient. Then you may have to take out all the sutures, which can be very difficult. That is another reason to be very careful in trying to reduce the incidence of suture cutting if you're using totally non-absorbable suture. I think that with a running suture you can significantly reduce not only the amount of astigmatism you get postoperatively—if you keep your wound fairly posterior—but particularly with mersilene, you can cut down somewhat on the amount of drift.

Simcoe: The closure that I use is a series of little double x's. I put the first bite in the sclera, then the next two bites across the incision—cornea, sclera, cornea, sclera—like a short shoelace. I come right back where I started. The last bite is cornea only, which buries the knot in the incision. At one time years ago, I used running sutures but had one that broke. I had a near disaster. I also like, if I have high cylinder, that I am able to remove one of those four little double-x sutures in the axis of the offending cylinder, and then the rest of the incision is secure. I don't remove one before seven or eight weeks, if I can help it. I'm personally a little afraid of trusting one suture the whole length of it, because the one that broke scared me to death.

QUESTION: Does the panel routinely use intraocular miotics?

Roberts: Yes, I routinely use intraocular miotics. My choice of miotic really depends on what I'm expecting in terms of postoperative intraocular pressure. For my routine patients I use acetylcholine; for patients with glaucoma or patients who for some other reason I expect are going to have high postoperative intraocular pressure, I use a stronger miotic. In that situation I use carbachol.

Balyeat: I use carbachol. After listening to Cal beat on me for a couple of days, I may change to acetylcholine.

Simcoe: I don't use miotics, but at one time I did. I got worried about the endothelium. It also seemed that some patients had more postoperative pain from the miosis, and maybe even inflammation from miosis. So, I dilate them with Mydriacyl and Neosynephrine preoperatively, and the pupils start coming down naturally that afternoon or that evening because Mydriacyl doesn't last all that long. I do give people acetazolamide postoperatively. I checked pressures at one time with it and without—that evening, nighttime, the next morning—and I found that for me the acetazolamide definitely made a difference. I didn't have those high pressure peaks. Do you have any experience with that?

Roberts: The whole key when giving acetazolamide is knowing when to give it. When do you give the first dose?

Simcoe: They get a dose preoperatively that morning, again following surgery, then that night and the next morning.

Roberts: If you're going to use it, the whole key is that you've got to use it early. I've spoken to several people who give people acetazolamide to take at bedtime after surgery. You're way too late then and miss the pressure spikes. If you're going to use it, then make sure that you give it preop or give it right after surgery. If we're going to do it, we have the nurse give it to them sometime before they leave from the ambulatory center to make sure they have it.

Simcoe: I agree. I tell them they may get a little numbness or tingling, but not to worry about it because it will go away in a couple of days when they quit. What about you?

Kalil: I use it, particularly in glaucoma patients.

Balyeat: I use it preoperatively one 500mg sequel, and I do it for the same reason. That is, not to reduce the pressure of the eye or the volume of the orbit or anything of that nature, but just to hopefully prevent the latent pressure spikes.

Simcoe: At the time I do the retrobulbar injection, I have the CRNA or anesthesiologist give a rapid intravenous bolus of mannitol, a 50cc bottle of the ¼% solution which is 12.5gm. That might seem like a homeopathic dose, but we give it. I read somewhere, years ago, that rapid injection has never caused anyone any trouble. I did a series of pressure readings with it and without it, and it distinctly has an effect on the pressure. If I'm operating on an eye and it's a controlled glaucoma, I will give them two vials. The neurosurgeons use multiples of that for their neurosurgery. One vial given rapidly I.V. generally works fine. I use two for a glaucoma patient, even when they're controlled. If the eye starts to get tense during surgery—I get a little worried about it—then I have them give another one and I wait a little while. It starts to act in seven or eight minutes and lasts a half hour, and for me, it works.

Roberts: Bill, some of this stuff is getting me a little bit concerned. We're dealing already with a geriatric population. In terms of PO medication or IV medication, your patients are getting diamox. They're getting systemic antibiotics. They're getting intravenous mannitol. Somebody is going to get sick from something. Mannitol scares the death out of me in an elderly patient. They could get Stevens-Johnson syndrome from the antibiotic, or they could vomit from the diamox and blow out their wound. I really think that our goal is trying to work on their eye, while doing as little as possible to affect their systemic health. So, we are not treating the doctor here; we're trying to treat the patient without affecting their systemic health.

Simcoe: I understand your point. The patients that we operate on, the geriatric patients, often are taking a dozen medicines anyway—they fill up the whole page. They're on all kinds of stuff and they seem to be getting by. If I were having trouble, I guarantee you that no one would have to tell me to stop. But I don't have any trouble. I have soft eyes to work on. I don't see any hypopyons anymore, and I don't have people with high pressures because I've checked them and I give them acetazolamide for a short time. So, as I've said, I'm not scientific; I don't really claim that; I know what works for me. When I compare what I'm doing now with what they were like before I did it, I can see a distinct difference. Does anybody else use mannitol preop?

Kalil: I have a little bit of experience with using mannitol intraoperatively. One thing to comment on is that when you give them a 50cc bolus, you're not dealing with the volume problems that you would if you hung up a 500cc bottle and ran it in. Also, it will work in 15 minutes or so. It takes maybe a little more time in my experience.

Simcoe: It's a peak effect.

Kalil: Right. And you do not get the problem of diuresis on the table because you haven't given them a large volume of fluid with it.

Simcoe: Have you hurt them or made them sick with it?

Kalil: No, not with the mannitol.

Simcoe: There were hands raised. Who uses mannitol? Do you have trouble with it?

Audience: No.

Simcoe: Does it help?

Audience: Yes.

QUESTION: Would the panel comment on what they consider a technique for adequate removal of viscoelastic.

Balyeat: My regimen is that if I'm doing a planned extracapsular operation, I use Healon. The main reason is that I use a manual cortical aspiration, and I find that Viscoat is particularly difficult to get out of the eye with a manual system. With an automated system, it's somewhat easier. But, I remove the Healon with the use of, in this case, a Gills-Welch cannula which seems to work fine. I do that before I start suturing. I then put in air which acts not only to keep the anterior chamber inflated, but it also irritates the iris a bit and at least I seem to get a little more miosis. One of the things the residents have a tendency to do is to leave the viscoelastic in the eye. They then inject an intraoperative miotic; but the pupil doesn't come down well, frequently because of the mechanical effects of the viscoelastic. I also don't like to be introducing a relatively large cannula into the eye after I've closed my wound. I can put in a 30 gauge needle then with balanced salt and replace the air. With phacoemulsification I use Viscoat because I am convinced that it does continue to coat the endothelium during the procedure. You can see the Viscoat there after the ultrasound. It is much more difficult to remove and I think one thing that will aid in the removal of Viscoat is to introduce some balanced salt solution with a cannula into the Viscoat. Sometimes the Viscoat will herniate spontaneously through the wound, but more often you have to use an automated I&A to remove it.

Roberts: I think there are two questions here. When you talk about removing the viscoelastic, are you removing the free viscoelastic, or are you removing the viscoelastic that is adherent into the trabecular meshwork? You shouldn't have a lot of trouble removing the free viscoelastic, especially if you are using Healon. Viscoat, as Hal said, has its own problem. The concern is the amount of hyaluronic acid that is adherent in the angle; that is what's causing the pressure rise. You can irrigate an awful lot and not get all the viscoelastic out. Just the fact that you use an adequate amount of irrigation, does not keep you from getting a pressure spike from the hyaluronic acid.

Simcoe: When I use viscoelastics, rarely, at the end I will use the little twin cannula that I use anyway doing the cortex, and many people have told me that it helps them to get it out.

QUESTION: During the workshop, Dr. Cooksey said that for dilating the pupil he uses viscous 10% Neosynephrine. Does any of the panel have experience with that?

Simcoe: I used it years ago, but I quit when there were two deaths reported in the literature from acute myocardial infection during hypertension crises as well as strokes in patients who received the 10%. It's so strong.

I was worried about that as a legal precedent. That's why I switched a long time ago to $2\frac{1}{2}$%. Some patients' blood pressures nearly went through the ceiling from the 10%.

QUESTION: Do the panelists who use the $2\frac{1}{2}$% find the blood pressure rises from that?

Balyeat: No.

Simcoe: Small and transient.

Balyeat: My experience has been that the pupils seem to stay relatively well dilated with the adrenaline, and I just haven't used anything else. Blood pressure elevation is a major problem. Of all the complications that I find in the elderly age group, it's the transient elevations of pressure that get quite high during a procedure. It certainly is nice to have those patients monitored and have either an anesthesiologist or CRNA to administer medication.

Chapter 17

PHACOEMULSIFICATION WORKSHOP

A STEP BY STEP APPROACH TO DOING PHACOEMULSIFICATION

As Presented at the New Orleans
Academy of Ophthalmology
John C. Cooksey, MD
Glen C. Cangelosi, MD

The following chapter will attempt to assimilate previous chapter discussions with the workshop held during the meeting and conducted by Dr. John Cooksey of Monroe, Louisiana. The intent of this chapter is to show an overall view of phacoemulsification without endorsing any particular technique. As the surgeon converts from extracapsular surgery to phacoemulsification, a variety of techniques should be known so that surgical maneuvers can be modified during any given procedure to accommodate the situation in that particular patient. Remember that phacoemulsification, like extracapsular extraction, is a procedure that builds upon itself. Each step prepares the surgeon for the next step. If you do one step wrong, it makes your next more difficult. With this in mind discussion of cataract extraction through the phacoemulsification technique shall begin.

After the patient is premedicated and placed on the operating table, intravenous methohexital sodium (Brevital) is given by the anesthesiologist to produce brief but complete patient amnesia. A retrobulbar/facial nerve or peribulbar block is administered using a 50:50 mixture of bupivacaine (Marcaine) and lidocaine (Xylocaine) in which 150 unit of hyaluronidase (Wydase) is added. An external pressure device is placed upon the eye if desired by the surgeon. The patient is then prepped and draped in the usual sterile fashion.

A lid speculum is put in place. A superior bridle suture is placed, if desired. Westcott scissors are used to perform a small peritomy, which is kept slightly larger than the anticipated incision size. A bipolar "eraser" type cautery is used to control any bleeding.

Incision

A caliper is set 1 mm larger than the optic width of the selected intraocular lens and the incision's length is marked at the surgical limbus. A half-depth ab-externo incision into the sclera is made 1–2 mm posterior to the surgical limbus and 1 mm longer than the intraocular lens diameter. This incision can be curved slightly parallelling the limbus or can be made as a straight incision but generally parallel to the limbus.

The second stage of the incision is the creation of a scleral pocket or partial thickness scleral flap. This incision is made with either a #69 Beaver blade or a Grieshaber Paufique knife. This incision is carried forward into clear cornea, creating a scleral-corneal shelf anterior to the base of the iris. This shelf creates a barrier that prevents iris prolapse during the remainder of the phacoemulsification procedure.

The third stage of the incision is the entry into the anterior chamber with a 3.1 mm keratome. This incision should also be made anteriorly to complete the corneoscleral shelf barrier.

It is not necessary to use a bridle suture, but if a bridle suture is used for the incision, it should be released at this point to maintain a deeper anterior chamber during the phacoemulsification and implantation of the intraocular lens.

A viscoelastic agent is instilled into the anterior chamber to maintain anterior chamber depth and to protect the corneal endothelium. A stab incision may be made in clear cornea near the 2 to 3 o'clock limbus with a #75 Beaver blade to be utilized later for a second instrument, if needed, during phacoemulsification.

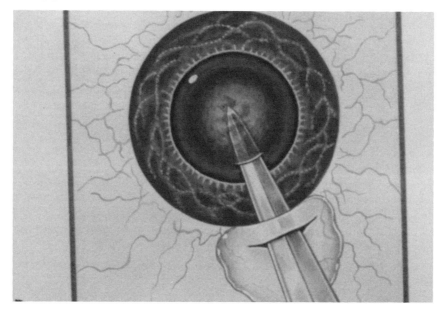

Figure 17-1:   3 mm Keratome used to enter anterior capsule parallel to pupillary border.

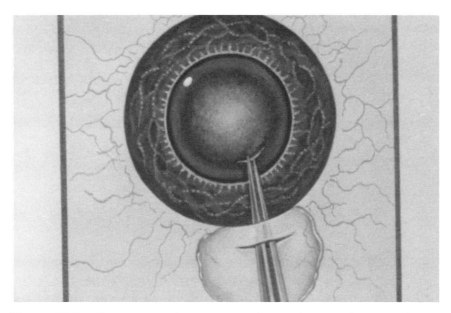

Figure 17-2: Forceps used to grasp and tear the anterior capsule.

Capsulotomy

Next a continuous tear circular capsulorhexis (CCC) is performed. This can be done by using either a prebent disposable needle or Utrata forceps. There are currently several ways of performing CCC being promoted, and the reader is referred to round table discussions and Dr. Gimbel's chapter on this technique. Continuous tear circular capsulorhexis can be per-

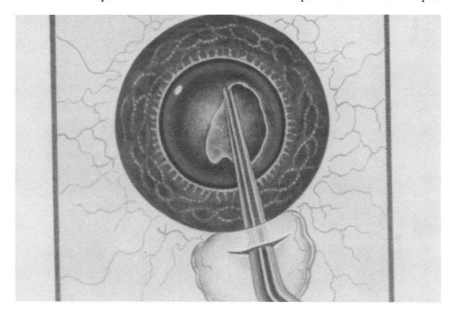

Figure 17-3: Capsulorhexis is continued towards 6 o'clock.

formed by using a 3 mm keratome to enter the anterior chamber through the scleral pocket incision. After entering the anterior chamber through this scleral pocket incision use the keratome to make an entry into the anterior capsule parallel to the pupil (Figure 17-1).

There are several points that should be made about the initial entry into the anterior capsule. First, this entry into the anterior capsule must be made so that the incision is a straight line incision that is parallel to the pupil just opposite the limbal incision. A radial incision in the anterior capsule will not tear properly. If the capsular incision ends up being a radial cut with the keratome, it should be converted to an incision that parallels the pupil by using a cystotome.

Once the incision is made parallel to the limbus and parallel to the pupil using the keratome, the Utratta capsular forceps or the Greishaber capsular forceps is used to tear the capsule (Figure 17-2). The capsule is grasped on the right side of the incision and the forceps is carried straight away from the 11 o'clock entry into the anterior chamber. The vector forces of the capsular forceps is toward 6 or 7 o'clock (Figure 17-3). The capsule will tear in an oval or round direction if the vector force of the forceps is carried first toward 7 o'clock and then turned slightly toward 6 o'clock (Figure 17-4). Once the 8 o'clock position is reached the capsule should best be regrasped and as the capsule is tearing through the 7 o'clock and then 6 o'clock position in a counter clockwise direction, the tear is turned further in a counter clockwise direction making it a round tear (Figures 17-5, 17-6, 17-7, 17-8, 17-9).

The best way to control the tear is to regrasp the capsule several times

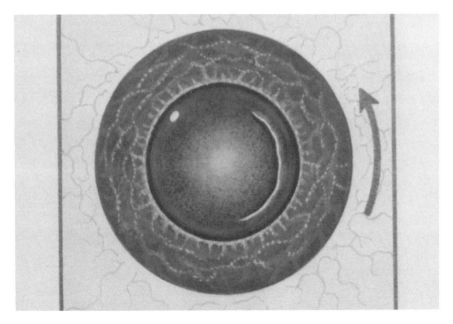

Figure 17-4: Desired direction of tear with forceps in initial movement.

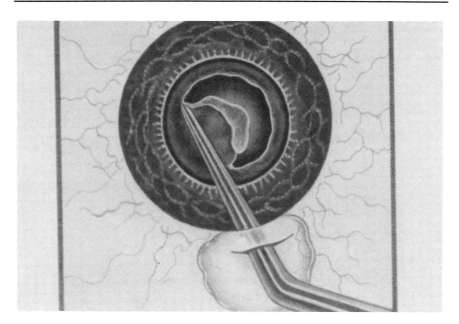

Figure 17-5: Capsule is regrasped at 6 o'clock and continued towards 9 o'clock.

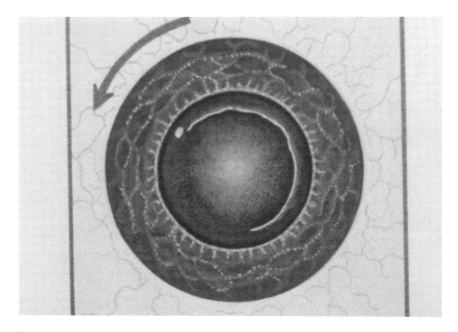

Figure 17-6: Desired direction and result following second manuever of tear.

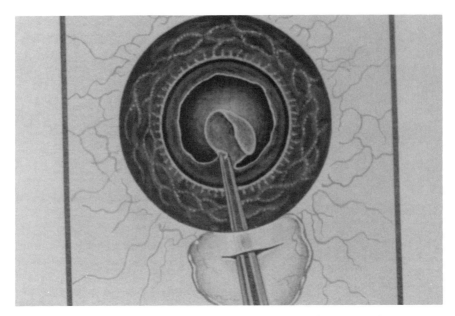

Figure 17-7: Capsule is regrasped for final tear towards 12 o'clock.

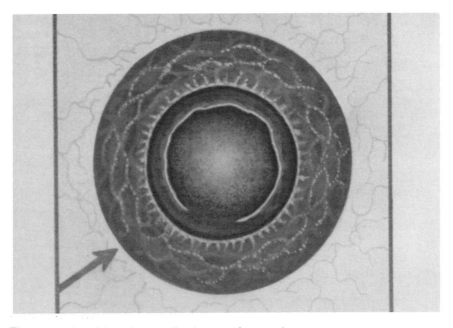

Figure 17-8: Direction of final tear of capsule.

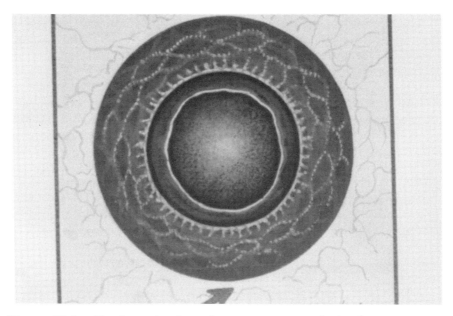

Figure 17-9:   Final result of continuous tear capsulorhexis.

at the edge of the tear. If you choose to only grasp the capsule approximately three times it is possible to complete a circular tear. However, you will find that as you go through the second half of the circle, you will be pulling the capsular flap in a direction that is almost 90 degrees to the desired direction of the tear. The more controlled method of making the tear capsulorhexis is to regrasp the capsular flap four or five times and holding it and pulling it in the desired direction of the tear.

This same technique can be carried out using a cystotome or bent 25 gauge needle. If the cystotome or the bent 25 gauge needle is used, it is important to fold the capsule so the pull is on a fold of the capsule.

In experienced hands, the cystotome and the bent needle seem to work as well as the capsular forceps in carrying out the circular capsular tear. It is, however, much easier to learn to do a circular capsular tear with capsular forceps than it is with the cystotome or the bent 25 gauge needle.

The size of the capsular tear, by the technique described, is determined by the initial incision in the capsule. If the initial incision into the capsule is near the pupil of the dilated iris (periphery of the capsule), the capsule will tear in a larger circle. In fact, the capsular tear is more likely to extend out toward the equator when a larger circular capsular tear is made. If the initial keratome incision of the capsule is closer to the center of the capsule, the capsular tear can end up being a very small circular capsular tear.

The initial keratome entry into the capsule should be approximately 1.5 mm or 2.0 mm within the pupil that is widely dilated to 8.0 mm. If the capsular tear is begun from this point the capsular opening will end up being 5 mm or 6 mm in diameter. The initial capsular entry should be approximately 3 mm from the optical axis or the optical center of the capsule.

The advantages of the continuous tear circular capsulorhexis are numerous. First, a circular tear will force the phacoemulsification surgeon to do the entire phacoemulsification procedure, or most of it, in the capsular bag and thus posterior to the plane of the iris preventing trauma to the corneal endothelium and the iris. As a corollary to this there is less fluid and lens turbulence when the emulsification is performed inside the small capsular opening. Secondly, the small circular capsular tear permits placement of the intraocular lens completely in the capsular bag. Thirdly, the circular capsular tear is a very resilient opening and will not tear radially the way a can opener type of capsulotomy tends to extend during the phacoemulsification or the lens implantation procedure.

There are certain trends that are evident in early 1990. The first trend is toward small incision phacoemulsification surgery. The second trend is toward circular tear capsulorhexis. The third trend is toward oval one-piece all PMMA intraocular lenses and foldable lenses. The continuous tear circular capsulorhexis compliments these other trends and also make us better phacoemulsification surgeons.

After capsulorhexis is complete, hydrodissection and hydrodelineation are performed. Without this step the phacoemulsification process is difficult. Balanced salt solution is gently injected between the anterior capsule and the nucleus towards the mid periphery of the lens until a fluid filled space between the nuclear and cortical zone is created. This is called a line of demarcation or demarcation zone (DMZ). This hydrodelineation step is followed by hydrodissection to completely dislocate the nucleus from the surrounding cortex. A prebent disposable 25 gauge irrigating needle can be used to hydrodelineate and dislocate/spin the nucleus in the bag.

Emulsification

There are many approaches to emulsification of the nucleus. There is no one technique that is perfect for every nucleus or for every surgeon.

This chapter classifies four approaches to emulsification:

1. Minimal lift
2. Endolenticular (capsular bag)
3. Bimanual
4. Endocapsular

Minimal Lift-Endolenticular

The minimal lift and endolenticular approach to the nucleus are essentially the same with two slight differences. The minimal lift technique is done through a larger capsulotomy and a good portion of the emulsification is done in the plane of the iris. The endolenticular technique is done entirely in the posterior chamber through a smaller capsulorhexis type opening.

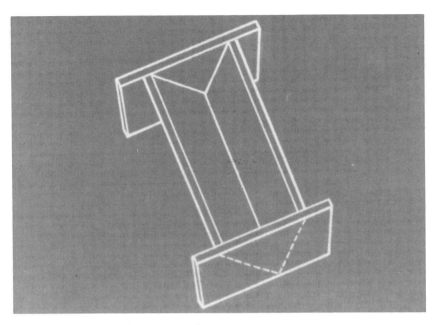

Figure 17-10: Imaginary trough.

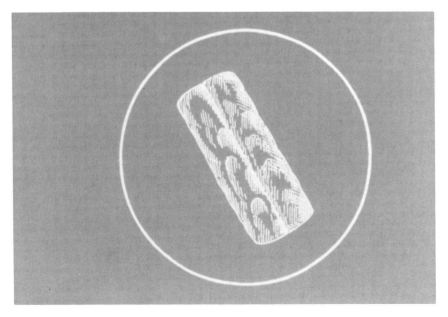

Figure 17-11: Phacoemulsification towards 5 o'clock creating a trough.

The minimal lift technique is a one-handed technique in which the nucleus moves anteriorly or upward as emulsification proceeds. The endolenticular technique is also a one-handed technique but the anterior capsular remnant of the smaller capsulorhexis holds the nucleus in the capsular bad as the nucleus is emulsified.

Beginning phacoemulsification surgeons should start with the minimal lift technique and progress to the endolenticular technique of emulsification as skill levels increase.

The excavation of the nucleus can be compared to three different eating dishes:

1. Trough
2. Bowl
3. Plate

The trough is the initial linear excavation in the 11 to 5 o'clock axis if the surgeon is right-handed and uses an 11 o'clock incision (Figure 17-10). Emulsify from 11 to 5 o'clock and create a trough shaped excavation (Figure 17-11). Use surgeon control. For a nucleus of an average density use a maximum power setting of 70%. Next enlarge the trough-shaped excavation to a bowl-shaped excavation. (Figure 17-12). This is done by sculpting each side of the trough and creating the bowl shaped, excavation of the nucleus (Figure 17-13). This creates the appearance of a doughnut in which the hole is not quite through and through.

The plate shaped nuclear remnant is created by taking the sides off of the "bowl" (Figure 17-14). The side is removed from the "bowl" by emul-

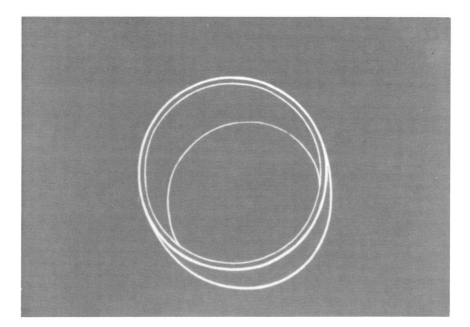

Figure 17-12:   Imaginary bowl-shaped excavation.

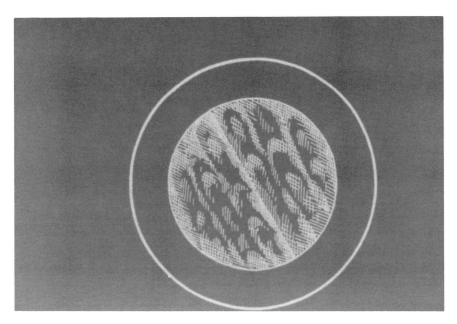

Figure 17-13: Phacoemulsification sculpturing to create a bowl-shaped excavation within the nucleus.

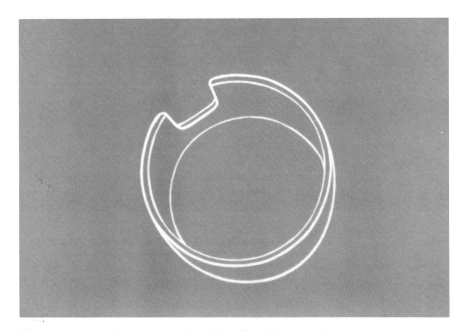

Figure 17-14: Removing the side off of the bowl.

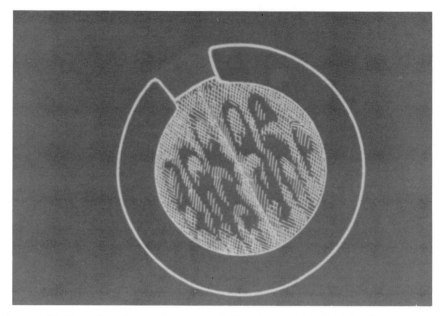

Figure 17-15: Continue phacoemulsification at the 5 o'clock periphery to take side off of the sculpted nucleus.

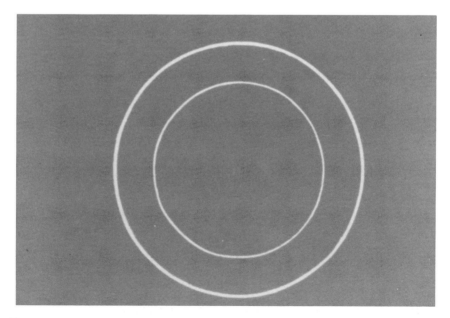

Figure 17-16: Imaginary "plate" remnant.

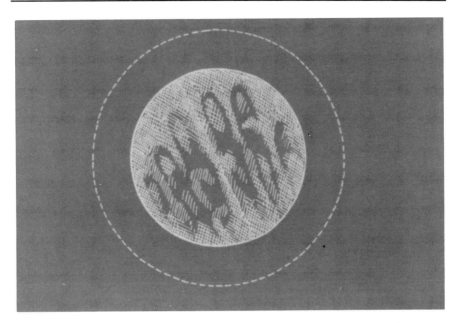

Figure 17-17: Phacoemulsify edge of bowl 360° to create nuclear "plate."

sifying at 5 o'clock to remove the equatorial portion of the nucleus (Figure 17-15). Once the 5 o'clock nucleus is removed, rotate the nucleus so that the 3 or 7 o'clock nucleus is in the 5 o'clock position. Again emulsify at 5 o'clock removing the equator of the nucleus. This process is carried out for 360 degrees until the entire equator of the nucleus is removed by emulsification leaving a plate shaped nuclear remnant (Figures 17-16 and 17-17).

The plate shaped nuclear remnant will rise to the plane of the iris and can be easily emulsified. Once the nucleus is reduced to a plate-shaped remnant it is usually possible to grasp an edge of the nucleus and quickly complete the emulsification.

The V-principle or trough cut should be kept in mind during the emulsification. The deeper that the excavation is made into the nucleus during the trough and bowl phase, the easier it will be to collapse the equator of the nucleus or the edge of the "bowl" into the center of the capsular bag.

Emulsify as deeply into the central nucleus as your skill level permits. Ideally a deep V or trough shaped cut is made up to but not through the posterior pole of the nucleus. The thinner the nucleus is centrally at the posterior pole, the more it will weaken the nucleus centrally and allow the equatorial nucleus to collapse into the central portion of the capsular bag where it is emulsified. This also improves the followability of the peripheral nucleus into the ultrasound tip. This is the same principle that Dr. Gimble and Dr. Sheppard are using with their cracking techniques.

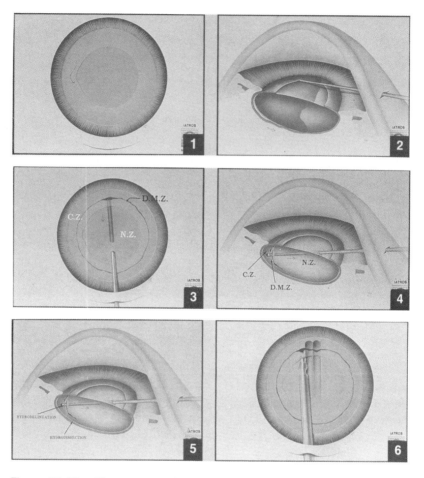

Figure 17-18: Phaco + step by step

1: Because of the small opening of the capsulorhexis, the approach to emulsifying the lens has changed radically. The Fractional ⅔ Phaco technique allows the surgeon to safely remove the lens from "inside-out" beginning at the center and emulsifying toward the periphery

2: Hydrodissection is used to form a fluid cleavage plane separating the capsule from its cortical attachments.

3 and 4: Hydrodelineation is used to separate the cataract into two concentric zones: the cortical zone and the nuclear zone. The ring of fluid that separates them is known as the demarcation zone (DMZ).

5: The combination of hydrodissection and hydrodelineation results in the cataract being divided into two concentric zones and isolated from the surrounding capsule. This approach reduces the chance of inadvertent capsular contact with the phaco tip.

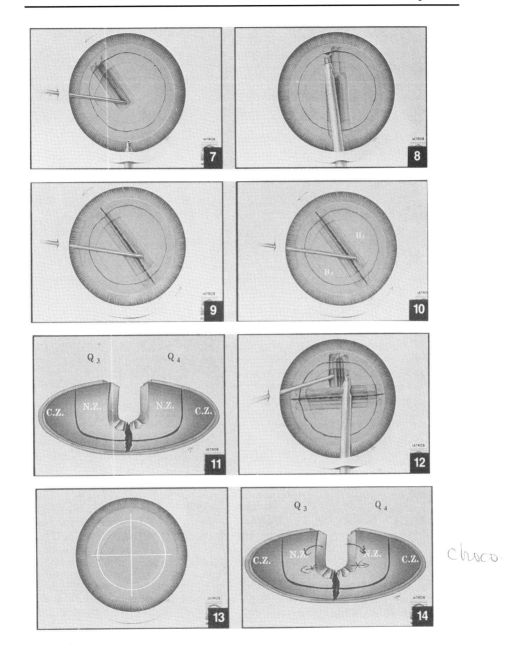

choco.

6, 7 and 8:   A central valley (CV), which tapers at the bottom to form a V, is sculpted in the lens.

9, 10 and 11:   The lens is then split into two halves (H1 and H2). Each half has already been divided into two zones: the nuclear zone (NZ) and cortical zone (CZ).

12, 13 and 14:   The nucleus is rotated 90° and further subdivided into two quarters. Again, each quarter has already been divided into nuclear and cortical zones.

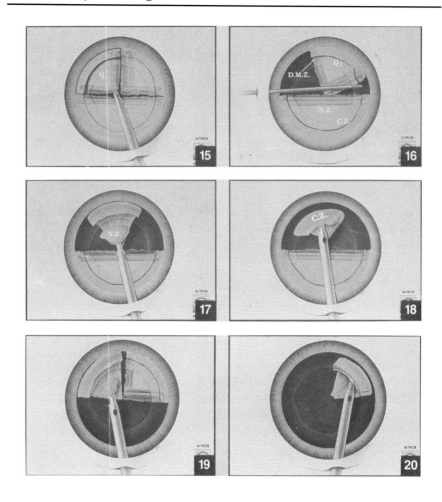

15, 16 and 17: Because the lens is now completely subdivided into two zones and into quarters, the path of least resistance for the first quarter is to simply follow the aspiration into the phaco tip without resistance. Notice that each quarter is removed in sequence—first the nuclear zone and then the cortical zone.

18, 19 and 20: The final half is again divided into quarters and each quarter is removed in sequence as before.

(This Figure has been reproduced with permission from OCULAR SURGERY NEWS, 8:5, March 1, 1990).

Shaving the nucleus is a good approach to emulsification. As you create the trough and the bowl, shave the nucleus in layers. Fill only 1/4 or 1/3 of the diameter of the ultrasound tip and thin out the layers of the nucleus. Shaving thin layers of nucleus is slower but safer.

By shaving with the ultrasound tip in an almost horizontal plane you are less likely to punch through the posterior capsule. Safety and control are particularly important to a beginning phacoemulsification surgeon.

Dr. Gimbel uses a cracking technique in which he bisects the nucleus and then emulsifies each half in the capsular bag behind a small capsulorhexis type capsulotomy (Figure 17-18). If you should decide to try this technique never use a large can opener type capsulotomy or the nucleus can get in front of the iris. When you bisect the nucleus only one half of it can be controlled during the emulsification phase. If the two halves are restrained within the capsular bag by capsulorhexis no damage can be done to the cornea.

There is a certain rhythm to be used when using the ultrasound tip while doing the initial sculpting of the nucleus. As you emulsify the anterior pole of the nucleus (creating the trough and the bowl), use high power at 11 o'clock and lower power at 5 o'clock. Start the cut into the nucleus as close to the peripheral edge of the capsulotomy at 11 o'clock as possible. Use a maximum power setting as you transverse across the optical axis and then reduce the power as the ultrasound tip reaches the 5 o'clock equator. Develop a power-on, power-off rhythm. Power on at 11 o'clock and power off at 5 o'clock. Use high power in the harder central portion of the nucleus. Use lower power at the posterior pole and the equator.

Use surgeon control to have greater control over the entire emulsification process. The mistake that many beginning phacoemulsification surgeons make is to put the ultrasound tip into the nucleus at 11 o'clock and then push on the nucleus without power until reaching the optical axis or mid-point of the nucleus. This puts undue and unnecessary stress on the zonules.

You can safely go up to 70% or even 100% power in this early phase of the emulsification. As you emulsify deeper into the nucleus approaching the posterior pole and the posterior capsule use a lower power setting.

Bimanual

The classic bimanual technique of phacoemulsification has been used by many good surgeons and had a place in the days of large can-opener capsulotomies. Today, with the use of small capsulorhexis capsulotomies there is less need for a bimanual technique. However, there will periodically be occasions when you need a second instrument in the eye and use it whenever necessary.

The classic bimanual technique is performed by sculpting out the central portion of the nucleus and creating an edge or shelf at 6 o'clock. The second instrument is then used to push downward toward 6 o'clock on the shelf of the nucleus and rotate the superior pole of the nucleus forward into the plane of the iris and into the anterior chamber.

The emulsification is carried out at 12 o'clock with the bimanual technique. This technique has the advantage of working on the edge of the nucleus which is faster than sculpting.

The two major disadvantages of the classic bimanual technique are:

1. Stress on the zonules at 6 o'clock.
2. Corneal contact with the nucleus in the plane of the iris and in the anterior chamber.

Familiarize yourself with the bimanual technique and use the second instrument if necessary.

Endocapsular

The Endocapsular technique of emulsification is done through an equatorial capsular opening on a soft nucleus. After the nucleus is emulsified and cortex removed the intraocular lens is implanted, and an anterior capsulotomy is performed.

With the present state of technology of phacoemulsification instrumentation and intraocular lenses there is no practical advantage to performing endocapsular surgery. When we have instrumentation that will permit efficient emulsification through a small equatorial capsulotomy, a safe chemical to prevent opacification of the capsule and an injectable material to fill and seal the capsular bag with optically precise lens material there will be a need for endocapsular phacoemulsification. This procedure represents the future.

Irrigation/Aspiration

Once the phacoemulsification step is accomplished, irrigation and aspiration are performed by either automated or manual techniques. Initial irrigation and aspiration of the 12 o'clock cortex may facilitate its removal since maneuverability through the small incision is limited and the remaining cortex within the rest of the bag can help maintain the bags shape during the procedure.

IOL Placement

After the I&A is performed, viscoelastic substance is introduced into the capsular bag and over the superior iris. The incision is widened to its full extent by a #75 blade. An implant of surgeon's preference is then placed into the capsular bag under direct visualization. If a traditional standard PMMA optic with haptics is used, the implant's optic can be grasped with Kelman-McPherson forceps in one hand and guided by the use of 0.12 forceps grasping the superior haptic with the other hand. The inferior loop is inserted into the inferior capsular bag. The superior haptic is then grasped with the Kelman-McPherson forceps. By a combination of bending the superior haptic and rotating the lens, the superior haptic is placed within the superior capsular bag. (If one is performing a small diameter

CCC and using a 14 mm length implant, capsular stress lines may be visualized during placement. Rotation of the implant at this time may produce a posterior capsular tear or rupture. The newly designed 12.5 mm diameter intraocular lenses may prevent this complication.)

Wound Closure

The viscoelastic substance is then aspirated and the pupil constricted with acetylcholine (Miochol). The wound is closed with the suture of the surgeon's preference with care in regards to its tension. It is often helpful to deepen the anterior chamber with BSS after placing but before tying the sutures. This helps in the estimation of the amount of tension to be placed on the wound as the sutures are tied. In this way excessive postoperative astigmatism may be avoided. A surgical keratometer can be used but may give variable results (see roundtable discussions).

One alternative method of closure is a "one stitch" variation. One stitch can be utilized to close the wound despite the use of 5 or 6 mm incision. To perform this stitch use a 11–0 mersilene on an Ethicon TG160–4 needle. First, take a bite through the scleral bed of the wound, horizontal to the incision. If you're right handed start on the right side of the incision; go through the scleral bed; come out and then regrasp the needle backhanded and place it through the underside of the scleral flap in the opposite direction, tying the knot within the wound.

The wound is then checked for leaks, the 6–0 silk suture removed and conjunctival flap pulled down over the wound site. Injectable gentamicin (Garamycin) 0.5cc and dexamethasone sodium (Decadron) 0.5cc can be given either subconjunctivally or presoaked in a 12 hour collagen shield placed over the cornea.

The goal of any surgeon should be to perform successful surgery rapidly, efficiently, and smoothly. However, the beginning phacoemulsification surgeons should remember that initial cases will probably take longer than extracapsular surgery and that patience is needed. Paying attention to detail and being flexible during surgery are invaluable virtues.

INDEX

Page numbers followed by t and f indicate tables and figures, respectively.